I0682737

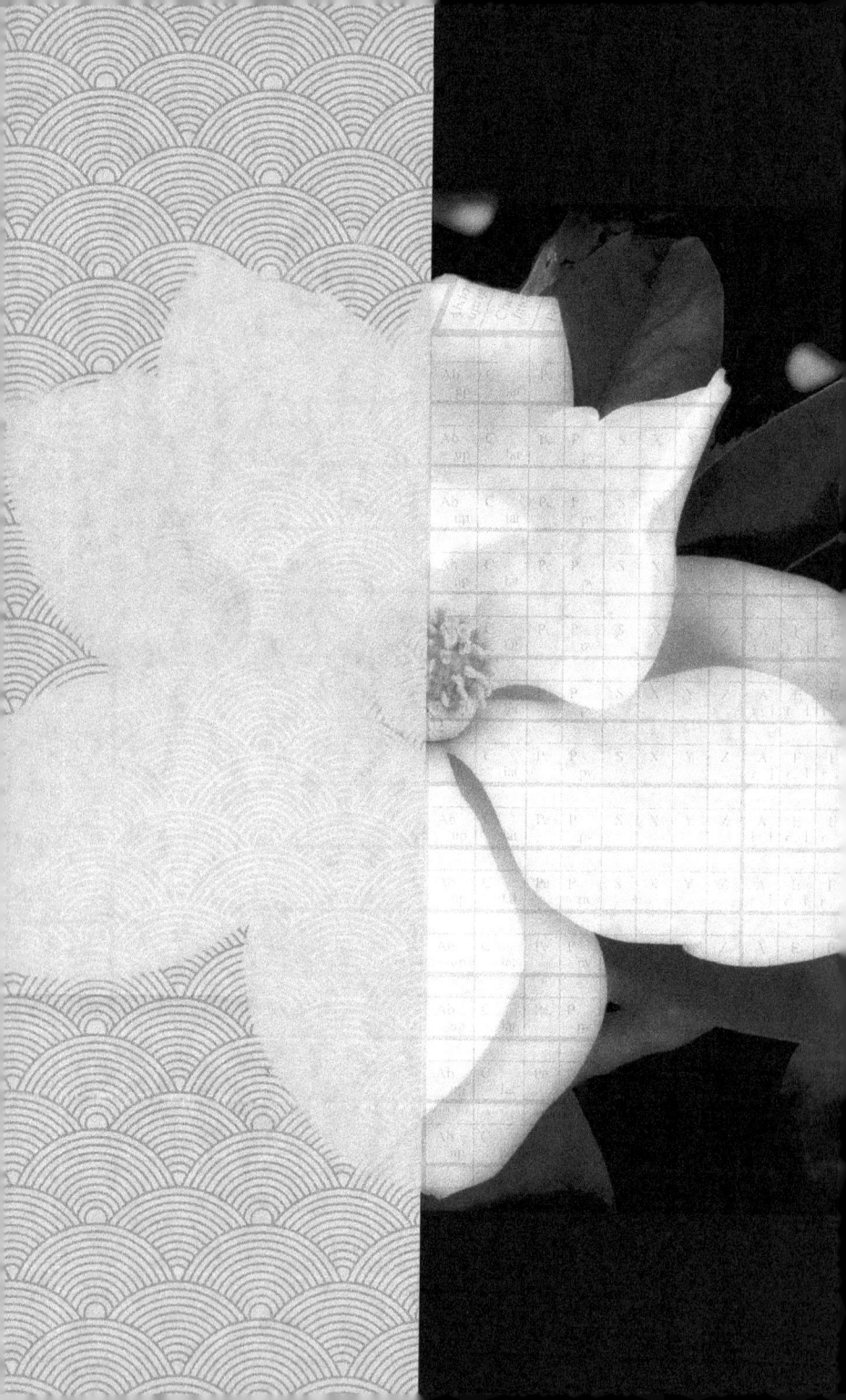

The Evolve Fertility Series

by Beth Alderman, MD, MPH

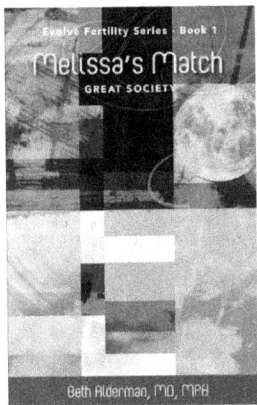

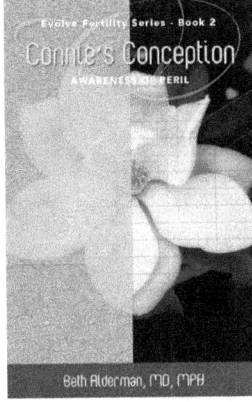

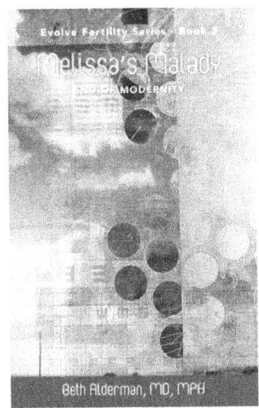

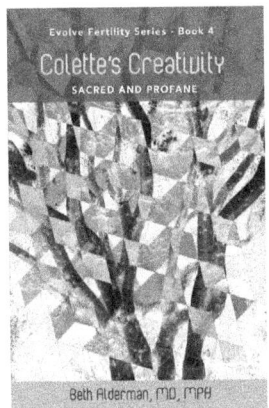

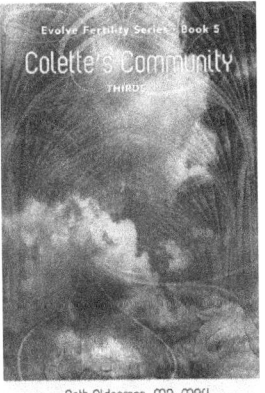

Connie's Conception

AWARENESS OF PERIL

Book Two of the
Evolve Fertility Series

Beth Alderman, MD, MPH

LIVING FUTURE BOOKS • ASHLAND, OREGON

Connie's Conception: Awareness of Peril
by Beth Alderman, MD, MPH
© 2019 FutureMedicine, LLC
www.LivingFutureBooks.com

For related online courses visit
www.LivingFutureCourses.com

All rights reserved. No part of this book may be used or reproduced by any means without the written permission of the author except in the case of brief quotations embodied in critical articles and reviews.

Editor: Julie Clayton
Cover Design: Bruce Bayard
Book Design: Book Savvy Studio

Library of Congress Control Number: 2019903850
ISBN: 978-1-7321110-0-4
First Edition
Printed in the United States of America

Contents

To Ellen

The most alarming of all man's assaults upon the environment is the contamination of air, earth, rivers, and sea with dangerous and even lethal minerals.

— RACHEL CARSON

1

Call for Aid

Connie's life has been sliding out of control for several weeks. Just as it is about to go into freefall, and she has decided to take a sick day to sort things out, her new protégé Dr. Gomez calls her for help. It is his first day of field work; Connie has never heard of an Epidemic Intelligence Service officer calling for help on the first day—or in the first week. She hangs up numbly, powers down her computer terminal, and stands up, which makes little difference to her height. At first glance, one might wonder if she is fierce because she is often overlooked, but that isn't it: she is always poised to fight injustice. She is also proud of her short stature and indigenous roots, of the pyramidal nose that looks Mayan but is Incan, the shiny black hair and the eyes that are light brown now because her pupils are tight with tension. She is beautiful but unapproachable in the way of a puma ready to pounce.

Just now, she is not sure whether she is tragical or comical. Inside she feels like a cartoon character crossing a fraying rope bridge that may at any moment cast her into the chasm where her demons lurk. Grabbing her packed travel bag, Connie barges out of her mildewed Atlanta office, barks instructions at an impassive ex-Marine squeezed behind the desk in the narrow corridor, and barrels out to the parking lot in the grip of a familiar, and therefore reassuring, righteous indignation. She is so worked up that she decides not to go home on her way to the airport. She doesn't want to take anything out on her beloved husband; she'll take things out on people she can't hurt—people who are far away.

Connie targets Dr. Parker Cowan, Chief of the Division of Birth Defects and Developmental Disabilities of the Centers for Disease Control, who accepted the rabbit-like Dr. Gomez as their Epidemic Intelligence Service officer over her objections. She even targets herself for allowing that mistake. But most of all, she targets Dr. Gomez. He didn't call for help from some Godforsaken place like Rwanda or Colombia—he called from Colorado, which has more resources than many nations of the world!

As Connie's car crawls along the congested, circuitous arterials of Atlanta in the tropical July heat, she feels a loss of hope. She doubts that the Centers will be able to do for chronic ailments what they did for infectious ones. The glory days when they were an integral part of the first-ever cure of the species—the eradication of smallpox—are gone. And the methods that still work for outbreaks of diarrhea and pneumonia and cholera and other familiar scourges do not work for these new problems.

She pulls herself back from the brink of despair by fueling her displeasure with Gomez. She first saw him during his new officer orientation where she had been sitting on the stage, simmering after a series of contentious meetings forced by budget cuts. Everything in the auditorum reinforced her distress, especially signs of lax maintenance like fingerprints on the brass flagpole and dust kittens clustered beneath the rows of hard wood seats. When her gaze fell on the giddy new officers, she saw only how the luster of ignorant optimism in their eyes would soon fade in the high-stakes world of field investigations; they would either win or fold depending on wit, likeability, and luck.

Her boss, the bony, thin-lipped Dr. Cowan whose bushy, strawberry-gray eyebrows reached all the way up to his former hairline, smiled benignly at the upturned faces and plodded cheerfully through circumlocutions designed to avoid upsetting the politicians several bureaucratic layers above—those anxious spirits who seemed to hover over the officers, waiting to pressure or dismiss anyone who failed to remain politically innocuous.

Connie's eyes had turned back to the audience and landed on the tall, lanky, beak-nosed Dr. Ramón Gomez. His full head of coarse black hair stuck straight up as if he'd slept on it. He looked up at Dr. Cowan with childish admiration, turned his big brown eyes to the woman next to him—a vapid-looking blonde with squashed features and a pushup bra—and raised his hand to ask naively, "What can we do to help?"

Given that all their problems were due to either political interference or institutional rigidity, Dr. Gomez' mindless compassion toward a malign bureaucracy struck her as dangerous. And now she has to spend hours on a plane and days in Denver—the last place she wants to go—in order to solve his problems.

When she arrives at Denver's Stapleton airport, Connie spots Gomez sitting behind the steering wheel of a rental car outside baggage claim. She's so tired that she merely plops herself into the car and grunts in greeting. As he drives them away, she sits with arms folded across her chest and barely registers the one-way streets that slice between rows of prosaic brick houses, watered-green lawns, and aging maples imported from distant woodlands. She feels as if a rocket engine is buzzing around inside her brain, and may at any point separate it from her body. She stops brooding only after Dr. Gomez zips through the commercial strip of Colorado Boulevard and pulls into a spot in a sunbaked patch of juniper-encircled asphalt. Sighing deeply, she relents a little. He's a safe and courteous driver, and doesn't waste words.

Connie jumps out into the thin dry air and follows Dr. Gomez into the atrium of an impressive new red brick and glass office building that seems to her a sign of boomtown overconfidence. After riding the elevator in silence, they enter a noisy third-floor suite labeled "Colorado Department of Health." A maze of spotless, carpet-covered cubicles with boxy desktop computers surrounds the glass-fronted office of the State Epidemiologist, Dr. Weinstein.

Connie enters Weinstein's office without knocking, plops down in a metal-edged chair, and fixes her eyes on his shiny forehead with the unblinking, disquieting stare that Dr. Cowan calls her predatory eye—a look that appears dangerous but is, in fact, a sign that her thoughts are elsewhere.

Dr. Weinstein, who is leaning back in his chair with a report on his lap, bolo strings trapped in his left armpit, cowboy boots propped on a white metal desk, looks up in surprise at the tiny brunette sitting in his office. She reminds him at first of a pretty, longhaired child in high heels; then, because of her rigid posture and dour expression, of a middle-aged patient with back pain. When Dr. Gomez sinks lightly into the empty seat beside her, Dr. Weinstein tosses aside his report and swings his feet down, sending his wheeled chair crashing into the filing cabinet behind him. Ignoring the reverberation of the hanging file drawers, he smiles boldly and leans over to shake Connie's hand, giving her a huge, toothy smile that she decides is equal in size to his forehead.

"Welcome, welcome, Dr. Martin, I can't tell you how much we appreciate you coming out on such short notice." Returning to his chair and leaning back once again, this time with his feet on the floor, Dr. Weinstein fixes his eyes above Connie's left ear and drawls, "Dr. Gomez here is doing a fine job, but we need someone with your experience for this particular press conference. Our little cluster has got itself blown way out of proportion. The public's hysterical, as always. We can't have that. You know what they say, the only fatality at Three Mile Island was that pregnant woman who panicked and crashed her car trying to get out of town. I'm sure you get the picture."

"I know what can happen in the absence of proper respect for public concerns."

Dr. Weinstein blinks as if hit by a stray spitball. The shock brings out his old Philly street persona, and with it the clipped style of speaking he's been trying hard to suppress since his arrival in Denver. "I'm sure I don't have to lecture you on the need for diplomacy."

Dr. Gomez frowns. He has heard that Connie is the bane of bureaucrats who get ahead by schmoozing, back-channeling, stroking egos, and otherwise massaging the system. She is also supposed to be the boon of people like him who put medicine, biology, and the well-being of all ahead of social status and money. She is said to be the best, which should include a good command of office politics.

Connie is pleased to have cut through Weinstein's infamous muck. She replies crisply, "We're here at the invitation of the State of Colorado and will, of course, defer to you in all aspects of the investigation."

Dr. Weinstein raises an eyebrow and looks at his watch. "Well then, as the CDC liaison in this state, I'm inviting you to meet with the key players at one o'clock. We need their buy-in before the press conference at four. Ramón's brought you up to speed?"

Connie frowns and crosses her legs. "Before we do anything, I want you to tell me your view of the rumors, case counts, medical records, denominator data—everything."

"I don't know any of that. You can have a look at what Ramón here put together for us."

Connie tries not to show her shock. Word has it that Weinstein is a blowhard. She'd never heard that he was incompetent. "Well, then, I'll need to see your press releases. I may have to backtrack before we can move forward."

"No backtracking. We can't afford to lose credibility. You ought to know better."

"I do. Do you have any credibility?"

Dr. Weinstein frowns before replying tartly, "Ramón can show you your desk. See you in thirty."

Dr. Gomez leads her to a carpeted cubicle with a desk, two chairs, bookshelves, a framed poster of a kitten hanging from a twig, and an ergonomic chair set far too high. Taking down the poster, Connie asks as she rolls it up, "Well, Ramón, what do you have?"

When she turns around to repeat the question, Connie notices a file folder open on the desk blotter with a box of hanging files beside it. Ramón, who is now sitting in the side chair, has just a hint of a smile in the crinkles around his huge brown eyes, which are focused on the folder.

Connie sits down to leaf through the exposed pages, noting aloud: "Six cases in Leadville in the first half of '86; three in Vail; five in Steamboat; two in Aspen; six in Alamosa; three in Telluride; two in Durango." After unfolding a map showing the case counts by county and pinning it above the desk, she unfolds another on which the counties are marked in four colors based on the proportion of births affected expressed as a count per 10,000 births. She pins that one up next to the first. "Hmph. No obvious pattern. Nice maps. What did you do before this?"

"I was a dysmorphology fellow at Hopkins."

"What do you think of the diagnostic classification of the cases?"

"If you'll allow me." Ramón, his face grave, stands and fishes a manila-covered medical record from the box and sets it on the blotter in front of Connie. Opening it to a picture of a newborn baby's face—or rather, what would have been the face had it not been split down the middle—he takes out his pocket pointer and traces the cleft. "The facial cleft is typical of the first cluster, severe but reparable. The hypertelorism is also characteristic, though in this baby, the index case, the eyes are particularly wide set. There's no side view, but a review of the medical record confirms that no external ears were found on physical exam."

"Any associated major birth defects?"

"No. A few cases have minor ones like umbilical hernia and digital reduction."

"Any family history or chromosomal anomalies?"

"No. One father with an isolated cleft lip; probably unrelated."

"What can you tell me about the pattern of defects?" Connie asks without missing a beat.

"It doesn't appear to fit a known syndrome. The dysmorphologists here are well-trained and experienced, and they've never seen anything like it."

"Are the Alamosa cases related to the Sangre de Cristos syndrome?"

"How did you— that hasn't been published yet! They swore me to secrecy!" Ramón exclaims.

"No, then?"

"It doesn't resemble any heritable defect reported from this region. Of course, even if it did, that probably wouldn't explain the new clusters."

"Perhaps. What is your assessment of the environmental hazards?"

"A lot of cases are from old mining towns with pervasive

hazards, so that could be a concern, but Alamosa doesn't fit the pattern, and the other areas are geologically heterogeneous."

"Do local environmentalists suspect anything?"

"Anything and everything: The naturally radioactive water in Coal Creek, contamination at Rocky Flats and the Arsenal, basements with high levels of radon, step-down transformers linked to leukemia. They worry about old mine shafts, mountains of mine debris, abandoned strip mines, an old tire depot that's been burning for years, and high carbon monoxide levels. To prove that any of these hazards causes any birth defect would be nearly impossible. All we can say with accuracy is that we don't know what we don't know."

"Good. No hint of a corporate cover-up?"

"No, certainly nothing like Chisso's attempt to cover up the connection between its mercury pollution and Minimata disease."

With Connie, people were either in or out, and Ramón was, to her very great surprise, near to being in. "I am surprised, Dr. Gomez, very much so. Excellent start. Why did you feel the need to call me?"

"I think that will become clear at the meeting."

"I beg your—Oh, well, all right, then. I'm here anyway. And the press releases?"

Ramón hadn't thought to collect them, but retrieves the file now. Upon reading them, Connie is so pleased with their non-committal vagueness that while she arrives at the meeting tardy, she is only barely annoyed at the prospect of yet another hour in bureaucratic purgatory. Frowning feebly at the grandiose table and lifeless faces, which she reads as reflecting the tedium of a complex and therefore self-absorbed organization—or perhaps the personal alienation of having become an institutional function—Connie tries to ignore Ira Weinstein, who is still too offended to resume his Western persona, and therefore did not save them seats.

Dr. Weinstein opens the meeting by introducing Connie and Ramón, then the others in attendance: The dysmorphologist from Children's Hospital, a lumpy, anxious woman in an out of season tweed suit; the Chief of the Environmental Division, a pale, laconic man in a pinstriped suit; the computer programmer, a trim young man in shirttails and jeans; and several others Connie doesn't bother to notice. She concludes that Dr. Weinstein has no more ability to identify key players than to plan a logical, practical, and transparent investigation. She is staring at the programmer with her predatory eye, trying to recall the embryology of facial clefts, when Dr. Weinstein adds in hushed tones, "Dr. Kazanjian, the surgeon, couldn't be with us, of course. His time is too valuable for meetings like this."

If anyone notices the implied insult, no blank or sycophantic expression shows any trace of it. The only reaction shown during Dr. Weinstein's significant pause is his own irritation at being interrupted by the breathless arrival of a plain looking, disheveled woman with a round face and brown hair. As her eyes scan the room for a free seat, she says breathlessly, "So sorry to be late, Ira, everybody, I took Colorado Boulevard and—" Suddenly she stops and gawps at Connie, then, half-laughing with astonishment, exclaims, "Pea? When did you get here? Cripes! Nobody tells me anything!"

"Missy?" Connie's eyes brighten and her expression opens. "Nobody told me either! Oh my God! I didn't recognize you! You've cut off your hair. And you've gotten so fat!"

No one misses the F word. The computer programmer grins boyishly, but the far plumper dysmorphologist looks horrified, and Ira Weinstein, whose girlfriend has trained him never to say such a thing, is shocked silent for a full five seconds, after which he breaks into a toothy grin in which Ramón sees triumph.

Ramón stares at Melissa in dread, but she only laughs and says, "Well, Pea, you haven't changed a bit!" Noticing the stares around the table, she rushes to take a seat, adding hastily in a stage whisper, "We should have coffee. Catch up."

Connie narrows her eyes and glances suspiciously at Ramón, whose poker face she can't read. Did he invite Connie to Colorado to expose her secrets, the ones Melissa knows? Her fears dissipate, though, as the meeting labors on and Dr. Weinstein reveals that he is effectively, although perhaps inadvertently, obstructing the investigation—not least by ignoring both Ramón, who is too junior to object, and Melissa, who represents an organization of parents, community physicians, and environmental groups, and who is therefore the only key player in the room. While Ramón probably invited Connie to neutralize Dr. Weinstein's interference, her first priority is to capitalize on the dumb luck that she and Melissa were friends in med school.

Dr. Weinstein intones, "People in the rural areas of this state don't care much for Denver until they need our help. Then they want us on their team, but they still want to do all the coaching." Connie looks impatiently at her watch and rolls her eyes at his whining—he is leaving her almost no time to write the press release. Then she sits up, open-mouthed as a realization strikes: Denver. Sports. With Dr. Weinstein having imbibed the local sports-mad gestalt, he could be a useful barometer of public opinion, able to communicate with the public in familiar metaphors. It is at this point that Connie decides she will bench him, not cut him.

When Dr. Weinstein leans back and puts his boots up on the table, which apparently signals the end of the meeting, Connie darts toward Melissa and grabs her elbow. "Can you spare a few minutes? We need your help."

"The press conference at the university, right? Um, sure. Tell you what, I'll drive you there on my way to pick up Dan for tonight's hike. We can talk in the car."

Ramón squeezes into the back seat of Melissa's tiny white four-cylinder, his head resting just inches from a smelly backpack. Clinging to the handle as the car squeals out of the parking lot and lurches into the flow of traffic on Colorado Boulevard, he leans forward, straining to hear over the breeze that is blowing through the open windows of Melissa's old, un-air-conditioned car.

"Personal chat later. Right now I need ten minutes on what's going on behind the scenes," Connie presses.

"Well, Weinstein's made himself pretty unpopular. He says the kids will be fine after surgery, and that these things happen. He even told a parent not to be hysterical. He isn't wrong, but he isn't right. He thinks everything's okay because the kids don't have a fatal defect, but you and I know, and he should know, that maternal-child bonding is tricky, and that very few mothers see past a defect like that quickly enough to bond at the critical time so as to be good parents down the line. And he should know that every pregnant woman in the state is terrified."

"Weinstein doesn't listen to you?"

"Well," Mclissa sighs. "It's like this: Ira's friends with my husband. You know the bolo and the cowboy boots? That's Ira emulating Dan, who is, like, the only Jewish hunter in the Rockies. So, when I try to talk to Ira, he imitates Dan not listening to me, and when I talk to Dan, Dan stonewalls me. I'm stuck. Absolutely stymied!"

Connie laughs. "And he tunes out the parents, too?"

"He's so out of touch! He blames the outbreak on inbreeding

11

in isolated mountain towns. Think about it. Vail wasn't even there thirty years ago. It has more people from South America than from Colorado. And the people there are completely obsessed with looks! You can't tell a mom with a nose job and tummy tuck that her kid is just fine without ears."

"And the environmentalists?"

"The upshot is that Weinstein doesn't see a likely cause, and again, he isn't wrong, but he doesn't acknowledge the fact that the science just isn't there. The only local risk factor that's been studied in any depth is high altitude, and the altitude hasn't changed lately. So ..." Melissa shrugs inconclusively.

She turns right abruptly, and speeds half a block further before screeching to a halt at the curb. Ramón opens the door and unfolds himself from the back seat before taking his bearings. The main entrance to the hospital is across the street; the disused classroom that Weinstein reserved for the press conference is in the building beside them.

Melissa fishes a card from her purse and hands it to Connie. "Call me. We've hardly talked lately!"

After Melissa speeds away, muffler rattling, Ramón leads Connie through the bare, shiny-surfaced hallways, shaking his arms loosely in an effort to relax. It doesn't work. He chose her in spite of her well-known rough edges because she is known for putting the patients and the public ahead of all else, and because their superiors are not free to do that. Either he underestimated her tension and overestimated his equanimity, or she is burning out, or his call was ill-timed in relation to the other investigations she is overseeing.

Ramón reminds himself that the people who dislike Connie most are often deeply envious as well, and speak of her work with grudging but nearly awestruck respect. She is the one Dr.

Cowan sends out to fix the mistakes of others: she wounds egos but saves reputations—and doesn't rely on the usual nervous but thorough application of known algorithms. She has, as her boss and mentor says, a rare sixth sense: an instinct for seeing through chaos and obfuscation, a knack for discovering what is out of kilter. Ramón is keen to absorb her art in the only way possible, through a kind of sub- or supra-conscious mimicry.

Ramón knows that Dr. Cowan uses Connie as the pet tiger in his back pocket, setting her loose to draw fire whenever he wants to cover his less-popular political maneuverings. Using her faults also puts Dr. Cowan in a position to use her talents. Ramón would admire Dr. Cowan more if he mended those faults as he exploited them, but Cowan is the most skillful strategist in the center, and Ramón is thrilled to have won this plum, if challenging, position.

So why are his shoulders hurting as they walk in silence through the maze of hallways? Something else is bothering him, something hidden. It must be doubt. It is always doubt, which is a perpetual problem for any scientist of faith. Science, especially something as uncertain as medical science, brings the mind into a state of skeptical questioning, while faith brings it into a state of confident calm. He is usually a little off balance in one direction or the other, but what is it that he is doubting now?

The answer comes to him immediately: He doubts Connie. In the complexity and confusion of a real investigation, the abstract ideas he wove together in the sheltered safety of the office and clinic are threatening to unravel. Why did she throw away Ira's goodwill before finding out anything about the investigation? What was it that the other Epidemic Intelligence Service and CDC officers said about him? Ramón can't recall. And why did she prefer the advice of the bumbling Melissa, who seems to exist only to irritate Ira at meetings?

Turning a corner, Ramón sees the door to the room where the press conference is to be held. Shaking his shoulders, he openly admits to Connie, "This is my first press conference."

"Then keep your mouth shut, and look like you know what you're doing."

Ramón is oddly comforted by Connie's blunt advice, which reminds him of how much he has yet to learn. Entering the plain classroom, he lengthens his pace and strides easily across it to the window, where he stands with legs apart and hands clasped behind him. Watching the sunlight play, he recalls his intention to heal the sick and slips into the Ignatian exercise based on Luke 8:22-25, where he visualizes himself steering the boat as Jesus calms the waters. He wants to embody that teaching now.

Connie's heels click as she hurries past the long narrow table at the front of the room to the far corner, where she sits down on a chair with a writing arm and takes out a pen and a pad of paper. Swinging her feet, which don't quite reach the floor, she stares at a pale, bandy-legged young man in frayed denims who is adjusting three white umbrella lights so that they will illuminate the front of the room. She doesn't notice the tiny dimples that appear in her pad of paper as she taps her pen absently, and allows her mind's eye to race over her previous press releases looking for one that will make a useful template.

His visualization finished, Ramón calmly takes a seat at the table and observes Connie closely. Minutes pass, and still she's written nothing. The reporters will be expecting a carefully prepared statement that reflects hours and hours of collective fretting over words like threat, hazard, and risk. Watching her reminds him of a bullfight he attended as a child, a bloody, protracted event that inflamed the impatient drunks in the sparse crowd and drew him in despite his horror. Now and then, the toreador had stood stock still even as the bull rushed at him, horns lowered. Ramón had felt part of the ritual slaughter— responsible, somehow, for the bull's death, and yet helpless to prevent it. He feels the same today: helpless, but calm. He can watch, and learn, regardless of whether Connie fails or prevails.

At four o'clock, when several staff members of the Department of Health, and nearly twenty members of the media have arrived, Ira and a few of his staff take seats behind the table. Connie jumps up to take the only remaining empty chair, turning into the blinding glare and heat of the lights. *This is it,* he thinks. *The hot seat.* When his eyes have adjusted to the milky light, he scans the faces of the reporters seated in the rows of student desks opposite. They look younger than he expected, and more cynical than hostile. Most hold pens or cassette recorders at the ready, a few fidget and whisper like primary school students.

Connie takes a micro-cassette recorder from her purse and sets it up in front of them as Ira begins, attempting his Western drawl— but, like most Hollywood actors, producing a Southern twang. "We've called you all here today to introduce Drs. Connie Martin and Ramón Gomez from the Centers for Disease Control—"

"Thank you so much, Dr. Weinstein, members of the press." Connie interrupts Ira in an earnest and dramatic tone; he nearly rebukes her, but catches himself and quietly sits down.

As Connie continues in a rush of words, "I will read a prepared statement, and then we will all take questions," she looks at the blank sheet of paper as if it is in fact a press release.

"The Colorado Department of Health has invited the Centers for Disease Control Division of Birth Defects and Developmental Disabilities to assist in its ongoing investigation of the clusters of facial cleft birth defects reported from several counties in recent months. We at the CDC have investigated birth defect clusters in many states and all over the world. We maintain a birth defects registry in Metropolitan Atlanta that can provide useful data for the purpose of risk estimation and statistical comparison. Dr. Cowan, head of our Division, has agreed to support the Colorado Department of Health team as requested by its manager Dr. Weinstein, and has committed his available staff and expertise."

Connie then puts down the piece of paper and looks directly at the television camera as she states: "After reviewing the data with Dr. Gomez today, I cannot confirm that your rates are higher than expected on the basis of chance alone, but I can confirm that the reported cases are very serious, and that their occurrence merits a full investigation, which we will continue to pursue. I cannot confirm any hazards to pregnant women or their unborn children, though we will be evaluating all potential hazards of concern to the public. Let me emphasize that such investigations may take many months to complete. During that time, anyone wishing to contact us with information or concerns should call Dr. Ramón Gomez at the Colorado Department of Health. He will issue periodic press statements to keep the public informed of our activities. As of today," she concludes, sliding the recorder toward Ira as if he were expecting it, "you can get copies of this statement from Dr. Weinstein. Questions?"

Ira stares at the recorder, befuddled, and then grabs it and thumps it into the hand of a mousy woman beside him, who takes it and leaves, presumably in search of a word processor and copy machine. Meantime, members of the press begin to ask questions that are savvier than Ramón expected, questions that are germane, precise, factual, and have practical implications—which means that they are not only worthwhile, but can be answered.

Then, with the few reporters who are actually hostile directing their questions to Ira, Ramón makes a mental note: Journalists who do their jobs well will make his job easier. He also knows he must stay calm in order to take in all of this so as to learn what he needs to know to master this field.

As Connie and Ramón make their way silently back to the street to find a cab, she fights discouragement of a kind she must hide, especially from Ramón. She doesn't like to cooperate with the pretenses inherent in societal conventions, in which are embedded so many lies, so much irresponsible conniving. She wonders if any of the soberly professional reporters who recorded her words understand that they are feeding the pervasive delusion that some individual or institution can protect the public health from the unknown, or from the fear of it.

Although she knows it is her job, and theirs, to control the panic, abet public denial and complacency, and shoulder the ambiguity and uncertainty, she doesn't like talking down to people as if they are children—and she doesn't like people escaping hard truths. While this collusive avoidance will sooner or later become untenable, and end in creeping nihilism or catastrophic loss of faith, at least no one invoked the devil, or shunned or murdered the unfortunate mothers or babies. As her thoughts turn to how things do improve, eventually, over the centuries, her spirits lift enough for her to feel hungry, and tired.

2
Nausea

✝

Six-thirty comes far too early. When the alarm rings across the room, Connie staggers out of bed and through her all-beige hotel bedroom into the all-beige bathroom. She lifts her nightgown over her head and frowns at the profile of her belly in the mirror. There is a definite bulge below her navel and her thighs are puffy.

I shouldn't be showing yet! But that's medical science for you, nothing but exceptions to fuzzy rules.

She looks down at the wastebasket under the sink and sees the blue tip of an indicator stick next to an empty pack of birth control pills. A wave of nausea rises, then retreats. Her next grievance reverberates loudly in the small room, "I hate these defects! I hate them! I hate them!"

But she must maintain. She can't spoil Ramón's careful planning by delaying the drive to Leadville.

Ten minutes later, Connie is dressed and made up and standing in the downstairs lobby, looking through the glass door of the hotel café. The bright lights and perky waitresses are too much for her, so she walks briskly out and down the cool street until she spots a tiny family restaurant with grimy windows. After darting in and sitting heavily on the most intact of the red-topped stools at the gray Formica counter, she turns her coffee cup right side up, nearly crying with relief when the matronly waitress greets her warmly in Spanish. Amongst strangers, she doesn't hesitate to use her legal name, Concepción Martín.

Connie wishes she could tell this woman everything. It would be so much easier to confess to a mother figure than a moribund priest, and in Spanish rather than English, but she knows that abortion is a not a topic for discussion. To Catholics, it is wrong, and that is that, whereas to her, it isn't so simple. It isn't simple at all. But she has to hold it together. She has to hold it all in because people are depending on her, as always: First her mother. Then her patients. Then her husband, who says his crazy computer games will make them rich at some undefined point in the future. And now her protégé Ramón, who yesterday revealed his true worth in his report to her; he is clearly a major new talent and so deserves her special attention for the sake of his future patients—people who are scattered among the community at large.

Connie orders *huevos rancheros,* of which she eats little, and limits her conversation to asking questions about family, giving her own personal recipe for an egg and lemon hair rinse, and requesting extra flour tortillas. She chews a dry tortilla, washes it down with sips of ice water, and thinks about her husband, who is undoubtedly at home in the den programming a new computer game and testing it at every opportunity. He will be eating, probably a wedge of the enchilada torte she left for him. Just thinking about him is deeply reassuring. He is her rock, or rather, her monolith. He is as tall and wide as she is short and slight, and is unfailingly placid, good-natured, and sweet. He delights in pleasures that come his way, but rarely finds a reason to leave the triangle formed by their bed, the computer, and the kitchen. He is his doctor's worst nightmare, but he is exactly as he wants to be, and Connie respects his choices.

"More coffee?" asks the short order cook, a withered,

unshaven man in a white hat who has come out from behind the grill.

"Oh, no thanks. Not today."

"You don't like the eggs?"

"I love the eggs! I'm just—a little nauseated."

"Would you like a roll? Some soda?" he asks solicitously.

"Yes, thanks," she replies, staring at her plate, mortified that he has seen through her.

As Connie takes a bite of the roll that appears in front of her, which calms her stomach, she overhears part of what seems to be a friendly argument.

"*Yo no puedo, yo no puedo,*" declares a sharp Argentine voice. "I'm getting my tubes tied!"

"You can't just give up on life like that!" counters a high-pitched voice.

"You've seen the pictures! They're monsters!"

Connie turns around to sneak a look at two young women in jeans who are sitting beside backpacks in a booth by the front window. She guesses that they are students on the way to a morning class at the nearby Auraria campus.

"How can you say that?" says the one with the high-pitched voice, a bleached blonde with big glasses looming over her empty plate. "They're helpless babies who need our love and support."

"If I had a child like that, I'd drown it, and then maybe kill myself," insists the Argentine theatrically. "In a few generations, we'll all be monsters! We've contaminated our food, our air, and our water, and we're doing nothing to stop it! What mother could bring a child into this crazy, suicidal world?"

Hearing her own secret fears tossed about sears Connie's mind and heart. She struggles to take it professionally, rather than personally. Her distress turns from hot to cold.

"But if you get your tubes tied, what happens when you meet the love of your life and he won't marry you because he wants kids?"

"Why would I want to marry someone like that? You make no sense!"

"You're the one that doesn't make any sense!"

Connie holds it in as she pays her bill, but when she passes their booth on her way out, she says coldly to the woman from South America, "If you had a baby, it would be most likely to die of injury."

"I beg your pardon!" declares the bleached blonde, placing her hand over her chest.

"Most infant deaths are due to injury. If you have a baby, buy a car seat." The Argentine shakes her stylish hairdo and laughs derisively, prompting Connie to tell her, in the rudest kind of Spanish, to go back to her mother's vagina.

That is the problem, Connie thinks as she leaves in a huff and charges up the street like a rhino. The arguments and counter-arguments are all absurd and, ultimately, beside the point. Ira was right—this cluster is taking up more than its fair share of psychic space. The tragedy of mis-birth had been broadcast, disseminated, magnified, and duplicated until a woman on the street believed that it made perfect sense to want to be sterilized.

But how will Connie make the right decision about her own pregnancy in this atmosphere of uncontrolled, unreasoning fear? She darts across the street to use a pay phone. "Hi Pip, honey, it's me!" Connie once called her husband pipsqueak, which stuck and evolved into Pip.

"Hiya, Pea," he replies, using the nickname Melissa made up years ago to tease Connie about being like the princess in the fairytale *The Princess and the Pea.* "What's all that noise?"

"I'm calling from a pay phone. Just wanted to say hi. So, um, are you lonely?"

"Of course, Pea," he replies, his mouth full of food. "I'm waiting (garble-garble) come home and (garble-garble) give me some of that Latin lovin.'"

"Oh, Pippie! You know, I've been thinking. Maybe we should use more protection. What if I got pregnant?" She wonders if he still feels the same as he did on their first date when, before their first kiss, they revealed the separate vows they had made never to have children. She is afraid to ask.

"Like you always say, how could you get pregnant on the pill?"

"I do say that, don't I?" Connie tenses and swallows. "Look, Pip, Hon, I may have to spend a lot of time here. Do you want your nephew to stay with you while I'm gone?"

"He's ten years old, Pea! What would he do while I worked?" Pip pauses, then asks with solemn intensity, "Pea? What's wrong?"

"I think I've seen one too many birth defects! Last night, I dreamt I was pregnant and I looked down at my belly and the baby's eyes moved together until they became one big eye, like those babies born with cyclopia in Cordobá, and then I pulled it out and it turned into a plastic doll and I lost it. It seemed so real! I couldn't sleep!"

"Pea, you don't have to do this kind of work. My new strategy game is almost ready to launch. Every kid in America will want one. We can already afford for you to stay home, and soon we'll have enough to get you a nice little practice."

Hearing the kindness and concern in his voice, Connie wants to nestle against his side, stroke his chest, and go back to sleep.

"You don't have to worry about me anymore, either," he continues. "I'm going to get my stomach stapled!"

At this, Connie begins to cry. "Oh, no!"

"I gotta stop eating! I want to be healthy for you!"

"Of couse, Hon. It's just that—you're my rock and I love you the way you are!"

"Will you love me thin?"

"Of course, my love. Always!"

"Pea? Pea, listen, I want you to come home as soon as possible. Okay?"

"Okay, Pippie," she sobs. "Okay."

3

House Call

✝

Connie thinks that she might recognize the house, a modest one-and-a-half story Victorian just beyond downtown Leadville. Painted a cheerful yellow, it has white trim and a tidy yard with a swing set in the back. She thinks the upper story might even have a view of the grand expanse of Mount Massive. But Leadville is shabbier than she remembers from dirving through here during her college days in Boulder, even a little desolate. But back when she was young, and poor, the very same home might have seemed enchanting.

Ramón parks, leads the way up the porch stairs, and knocks politely as Connie tries to look through the bevel-edged oval window in the heavy front door. She can see nothing of the dark interior through the sheer curtains. Shortly, a woman with a freckled nose and deep-set eyes opens the door, greeting Ramón warmly while looking Connie up and down warily.

"Hello, Mrs. Schultz," Connie says, using the authoritative and funereal voice she deploys when giving Bad News to moms. "I'm Dr. Connie Martin with the CDC. Thank you for agreeing to talk with Dr. Gomez and me today. May I see the patient now?"

Patty Schultz motions them into the front parlor, which is full of heavy oak antiques adorned with Victorian lace. Several twenty- to thirty-year-old women are sitting in a ragged circle on old misshapen cushions, reminding Connie of a vigil. The room resembles her first landlady's parlor so much that she can almost hear a quavering voice scolding her for running. Straightening up as tall as possible in her high-heeled sandals, she intends to put the group at ease, but only manages a stuffy, "How do you all do on this fine day?" Ramón puts on his poker face in preparation for further *faux pas*.

"Hi, I'm Sally with Colorado Parents for Healthy Babies," says a long-faced woman in cycling shorts and a jogging shirt, her words accelerating like a bicycle going downhill. "Liz and Jill had babies like Patty's, and the rest of us are moms, too, and we want to know when you're going to do something about this!"

"Have you talked with Dr. Weinstein?" Connie asks strategically.

Sally leans forward and begins passionately, "Yes! He's been a real—"

When Patty interjects sharply, "We're glad Dr. Gomez and you have come out to help," Sally closes her mouth and folds her arms.

Patty then motions to Connie and says, "Come on back." As they walk down a long hallway, Connie notices a decorative pair of gut-strung wooden snowshoes, an X formed by a pair of brand new metal ice axes, and a utility rack full of long skis of varying widths and bindings hanging on one wall. At the end of the hall, they enter a tiny, pale green nursery and slowly approach a wooden crib decorated with yellow floral bumpers and ruffles. Suspended above the crib is a black design on a white circle that mimics the instinctively recognizable pattern of a human face.

Looking over the edge of the crib, Patty holds a finger to her lips, then circles to the opposite side and motions for Connie to approach. Placing her hands on the near rail, Connie peers down at a baby sleeping on his back, elbows and knees bent at right angles with his face toward her. She has never seen a cleft this severe in a viable fetus, much less a living child. It looks as if a surgeon had made a deep but bloodless midline cut from the baby's brow to his lower lip and all the way through his palate, which Connie glimpses through the cleft in the upper lip. Upset at seeing little formative tissue in the deep and wide gap, she knows a surgeon may have little to work with. Severe and lasting disfigurement is likely. She tries to estimate the chances of developmental delays.

As Patty watches her son sleep, her hands folded tightly on top of the opposite rail, Connie whispers softly, invoking one of Dr. Cowan's stock phrases.

"Every time I see a child like this, I remember how infinitely complex new life always is, how it's never perfect, how survival is always perilous and miraculous, no matter how much we take it for granted." She likes to remind mothers, and herself, to feel more grateful and less ashamed. It is essential to rally their spirits for the sake of the baby.

While watching the sleeping innocent, though, she thinks of the pain he will endure in his first surgery alone, and reaches out impulsively to pick him up. Resting him carefully on her shoulder, where he fusses and then settles, she continues in a broken voice, "How tragic that your baby's beauty should be so hidden, that he should have to suffer so much pain!" Connie is genuinely teary-eyed. "I don't know how you can handle this—wound!"

Patty's fingers tighten until her knuckles turn white, but her voice remains calm. "It's easier for me than for some. I already have a normal son. It's harder if it's your first. And I have a sister who went blind when we were small, from meningitis. I used to play with her in the dark, or blindfolded. So, when I had Hector, I just closed my eyes and pretended to see him the way she would."

Connie closes her eyes and feels his warmth, his weight,

and the moisture from his mouth, which is soaking through the shoulder of her two-piece cotton dress. He feels helpless, trusting, contented. "Yes! It's much easier to see him properly this way."

When Hector fusses again, Patty releases her grip on the rail, and her hands fly toward him. Connie hands the baby carefully, supporting the fragile stem of his neck. "My mother always used to say that babies are sent to test us, but I think maybe some babies, like this baby, find the right mother. Tell me, though, why did you put off the surgery? I can see that he's growing well, but how is he able to eat?"

"We're waiting for the cartilage to grow. He can take the breast."

"A good choice, but a hard one. I'm surprised the surgeon suggested it."

"He didn't. Dr. Kazanjian wasn't—well, he listened eventually. We can make the tough choices in this family. You have kids?"

"No." Connie turns and walks briskly back down the hall.

Ramón feels a shock of embarrassment on seeing the mascara-outlined tear tracks on Connie's cheeks. He is sure that Patty, who enters with Hector in her arms, must disapprove of this unprofessional behavior.

But the women in the room seem to have come to some kind of invisible understanding in Connie's favor. As he and Connie walk out to the car, Patty waves from the doorway and calls out, "Whatever you need, just let us know." Ramón is dumbfounded.

After waving back, Connie hops into her seat and slumps down, preoccupied. Her mind seems to have split in two: One half is dwelling on the miraculous blessing of conception and birth, and the other on the horror of failure. The tiniest alteration in the division of a single cell can make the difference between life and death, between sublimity and suffering. Any mishap early in gestation could have devastating consequences. The idea that any part of development might be random is ridiculous. But people want statistics, and that's what she'll give them. She has no choice. Ramón too gets in the car, then pauses a moment, hands on the steering wheel. He ventures gently, "I thought they might be upset by tears. I suppose that's how us men think."

"No one's on their side. Not really. Everyone thinks that the unknown is someone else's problem. If we drop the ball, there's no one to pick it up. It isn't right."

The silence afterward is tense. Descriptions of Connie had included words like indestructible, tough, and mean. No one used the word high-strung, but she reminds him of his little sister as a tense, brittle teenager—always crying, picking at her food, and taking offense at casual comments.

He thought back to the drive up from Denver, when she had frustrated his every attempt to get to know her. "So, Connie, where are you from?"

Her reply had been evasive. "I've spent time in so many places that I feel like I'm from nowhere and everywhere!"

"I grew up in Chicago, but I was born in Puerto Rico," he'd said. "I don't remember much about it, just the heat in the summer, and the wonderful times when my father drove us to the beach to cool off."

When Connie made no reply, Ramón tried a series of topics, starting with the scenery and the weather, then moving on to music, family, sports, politics, and travel. Finally, he got Connie onto the topic of computer games, about which she was remarkably knowledgeable. She had continued with a long monologue about the benefits of programming in C++, after which he had been relieved to ride the rest of the way in silence.

As Ramón pulls away from the curb and into the pale, bright

sunlight, he almost gasps as the silences then and now click into place. Of course! Connie is hiding something, probably something to do with birth defects! Doctors who specialize in oncology have often lost a loved one to cancer; Connie probably came from a family with a history of birth defects, a history hidden in secrecy and shame.

He should have thought of that earlier, especially as his own family was like that. Ramón was only ten when his little nephew, whose birth had been so anxiously awaited, was locked away behind a heavy door to die alone. Although Ramón had heard whispers about his nephew being born a monster, he had been forbidden to talk about it with anyone, including his sister. He had reluctantly obeyed, but from that moment had resolved to become a doctor who would find out what caused babies to turn into monsters, and to make sure that it never happened again.

"Stop! Stop!" Connie shouts suddenly, pulling at the door handle in agitation.

Ramón slams on the brakes reflexively, but before he can pull up to the curb, Connie jumps out of the car and runs between two tiny but tidy wood frame houses on treeless lots, shouting, "Stop him!"

Connie had spotted a small group of young children playing in what appeared to be a pile of dirt. It was only a block from the Schultz home, yet near enough to the far end of town that it backed onto a huge mound that Connie recognized as tailings from a nearby mine. One of the children was eating what at first glance seemed to be dirt, but which must be pulverized lead ore. By the time she reaches the children, they have scattered in all directions, leaving only a toddler who is standing still, clutching his bottle and crying as he rubs tailings on his face.

"No, don't!" Connie yells frantically.

"Get away from my son!"

As Connie turns to see a stocky, muscular woman running toward the toddler in alarm, she exclaims, "He was eating the tailings! He'll have to be tested for lead!"

"Who the hell are you?" The woman snatches up the toddler and holds him away from Connie, who is, up close, not at all threatening.

"I'm Dr. Martin of the Centers for Disease Control. We just left Patty's house, and I saw your son eating this lead ore!"

The woman looks at her in amazement and then bursts into laughter. "Of course he was. They all do. You outsiders! Always interfering."

Connie is tempted to scold this idiotic woman, who evidently thinks it is fine for her child to eat mine tailings that everyone knows could poison his brain, but she can see that the mother believes what she is saying. Looking from the mother to the tailings pile in the yard, which supports only a few bunches of crabgrass, Connie asks, "Would it be all right if we took some samples to the lab? Just to be sure."

Ramón appears behind Connie, panting in the thin air. "Is everything all right?"

"Yes," Connie replies. "I just saw this young fellow eating tailings and wanted to be sure he was all right."

"Would it be okay with you if we took some samples?" Ramón repeats anxiously.

The toddler squirms, folding himself forward and then arching back as if to make a swan dive. The woman grabs him protectively and turns back to the house, muttering over her shoulder, "Suit yourself."

They hadn't come prepared to collect environmental samples. The only acceptable container Ramón finds in his bag is a stool specimen jar, which he uses to scrape off a sample of the gray, gritty mountain of waste. Capping it awkwardly as they walk back to the car in silence, he realizes that they are both galvanized into a tense state of suspicion and determination.

Connie has been skeptical about some of the local environmentalist's concerns that are being reported to the Department of Health, most of which reflect vague or inaccurate notions of biology—and are muddied by resentment or fear. One letter writer came right out and said that he hoped to use the afflicted children to "get" a polluter, an abuse of misfortune that Connie finds reprehensible. She has suspected that the activists will be nothing more than obstacles and irritants, but the disturbing sight of a toddler eating lead ore has altered her view. Her censure of neglectful mothers alloys with her contempt for opportunists into a cold, hard determination to identify the guilty hazards.

Ramón resumes his course on the road leading north out of town, glad that he already arranged to follow up on a concern about the Climax Mine. It was raised in an articulate and persuasive letter from a member of the local Sierra Club who was also a professor emeritus at the Colorado School of Mines. Although the professor's biological rationale made little sense, his environmental rationale was solid. Ramón was impressed by the man's credentials as an expert in hydrology, and the connection he made between the mine and local drinking water—which could potentially affect the health of the unborn.

Connie is pleased that Ramón was so perspicacious as to arrange this visit. She also wonders if he knows more than he is letting on. She would ordinarily take comfort from that thought, and from the familiar scenery, especially after they turn onto a road that forks to the right through a spectacular high valley. But she is far too nauseated, which she tries to hide by feigning sleep.

When Ramón gently calls to her, Connie opens her eyes again and wonders, momentarily, if she is having a nightmare that the planet has become a barren wasteland. Their surroundings resemble pictures sent back by a lunar lander, although the mountains are too high and steep and angular, and there is too much color. Accenting the predominantly gray tones are purples and greens that lurk deep in the shadows of the tailings and the rain-heavy afternoon clouds that are flying over the ridge to the north and west. Connie has never seen a strip mine up close, and the impact is like a death: awful, incomprehensible, inescapable. It is greed, not faith, that moves mountains—greed that sterilizes the Earth and makes it unfit for new life.

Ramón too is horrified at the sight of the glorious creation of God having given way to a kind of mineral holocaust. He never liked the industrial areas of Chicago, where he moved with his family when he was six. Back then, he tried to tell himself that without industry there would be no El to take him to school; no flights to take him home to Puerto Rico; no heat to keep out the bitter winters; no transport system to bring him beans and rice; no job for his father. But now he remembers their vast and inhuman installations spreading out like a hungry maw, to eat the Earth, too slow to be frightening, and too idolized to be recognized as the Gog and Magog of a coming End Time.

In retrospect, he believes that he saw this very young, as a revelation, as proof that God is still speaking. But he had been too young to articulate it properly, and his words had gone unheeded. In the end, his only choice was to block it all out. But he can't block out this devastation. Nor can he take it in.

"Keep going," Connie directs. The sight of overwhelming destruction has made her feel protective of Ramón, and after a series of hairpin turns she points to a gravel road.

"Turn here!"

Ramón swerves onto a flat stretch of road, stopping before it ascends out of sight behind the nearest and smallest tailings pile. Looking past a hundred-foot heap of gray-white rubble on their right, Connie suddenly points out her window.

"Look at that run-off! It's like soylent green!"

She jumps out of the car, scuffs over to the edge of the road's shoulder, and leans out for a better view. Ramón follows, stepping carefully and toeing clods of earth before peering down a steep, twenty-foot slope that bottoms out into a pool of opaque, neon green water. Connie folds her arms and sighs in exasperation. "Everyone always thinks it's the water. But it's never the water!"

"Remember the Eagle-Vail training exercise?" Ramón asks evenly. "The one we do the first week of EIS training? It's based on an outbreak of gastrointestinal disease in Vail that resulted from a failure of sewage treatment upstream."

"Well, yes, infectious diseases. But birth defects? Even if we knew that something in this ..." Connie makes a sour face, "... this swill, could cause birth defects of any kind, how would that something get from here into the drinking water of pregnant women in Leadville?"

"We're just below the Continental Divide here, at the headwaters of the East Fork of the Arkansas River, which flows through Leadville some thirteen miles downstream."

"Yes, but this wouldn't flow directly into anyone's tap, not without the knowledge of the Health Department, which monitors the quality of Leadville's municipal water supply."

"There could be surges or run-off between sampling times. We could ask case mothers about their sources of drinking water."

"Yes, well, that would be prudent, but—" Connie's memory moves in like a zoom lens on the objects hanging in Patty's hall.

"Some of these women may be outdoors people. Patty had skis, snowshoes, everything. She might have drunk surface water. What, exactly, did that hydrologist have to say?"

Ramón lopes back to the car and retrieves the letter from his shoulder bag, panting as he returns. Connie takes it and begins to read, "… possibility of storm run-off … drinking water quality checked infrequently … uncertainty about underground water flow … hmph. Yes, all right. Let's take a sample of that swill. Find out what's in it." She holds the letter out to Ramón and crosses her arms again.

Ramón, who is by no means fond of heights or nimble at altitude, walks slowly back to the car in search of something they can use to hold a water sample. Then, making his way gingerly down the slippery tailings, he loses his footing in the last eight feet, slides the rest of the way, bracing himself with his right hand to avoid a fall. Finally, at the bottom, he squats at the edge of the water and scoops a few ounces of the suspicious looking liquid into an empty spring water bottle that until recently had been rolling around on the floor of the car.

As he scales the slippery slope, bottle in hand, he feels a strange sense of excitement that is half dread at the thought of water poisoned on a massive and irremediable scale, and half elation at the possibility of uncovering the elusive cause of the defects—thereby pointing the way to mending the sins of his species, which fall most heavily on the unborn and the youngest.

4

Legacy

✝

During the long ride back to Denver, the magnificent peaks seem but a craggy obstacle to the car that struggles over the passes like a tired, unresponsive horse. When they finally reach the low-rise brick complex of the Health Sciences Center, Connie jumps out, slinging her bag over her shoulder. Staggering to keep her balance, she hurries away to find the environmental scientist whom Dr. Ira Weinstein recommended. Ramón continues on toward Loveland, already late for a meeting with the veterinarian who delivered a two-headed calf that is worrying families in the surrounding counties.

Connie shares their fears. After seeing the lime green water beyond Leadville, she feels tense and suspicious, and so distracted that she has to ask for directions several times before finding Dr. Vanier's laboratory—which is distinguished only by the number on a tiny plaque above the door. The interior is crammed with apparatuses, from a series of flasks for distillation to an assortment of gray metal boxes, one of which Connie recognizes as a spectrophotometer.

Connie's eye is soon drawn to a repetitive pattern of concentric ovals that look like thick, multicolored isobars with jagged edges. Approaching, she sees that it is the display on an oversized monitor attached to a large, metal computer box. Behind it, a wall poster that seems to show a three-dimensional view of the same pattern turns out to be a panorama of the Rocky Mountains from space reconstructed from Landsat images. Next to the monitor, a dot matrix printer starts up with a sound like a table saw and begins spitting out a roll of paper with fourfold tables produced by a familiar statistical software package for micro-computers.

"Hello?"

Connie turns to see a trim young man wearing a bicycle helmet, a light blue shirt with a button-down collar, and chino pants that he has bound around the ankles with reflective strips. Before she can reply, she hears a creaking sound ending in the word "Eureka!" and looks up to see a huge white cockatoo perched on a branch above one of the many metal boxes lining the wall. He tips his head and stares down at her with one unblinking eye.

"Do you hear that a lot around here?" Connie asks.

The man looks at her skeptically for a moment, and then carefully arranges his face into an expression of patient acceptance. "May I help you?"

"Eureka! Eureka! Eureka!"

"I'm Dr. Connie Martin for Professor Vanier. Is he here? Is this yours?"

"Isaiah's his bird, so if the parrot's here, Dr. Vanier's here, too."

"No, I mean, is this picture yours? Is it a screen saver?"

The man looks at her penetratingly for what seems a long time, and then replies hesitantly, as if it were a secret, "Yes, it's mine, but it isn't a screen saver."

"What is it, then? You're printing out the usual statistics, but this looks like a sci-fi prop, or part of a Navajo weaving."

He passes his hand over the display as if petting it and replies, "It's a display that I devised in order to look for patterns in the data."

"Data dredging! Isn't that a bit like reading tea leaves?"

"Tables and indices sometimes hide things that the eye can

perceive." He sits on one of the old oaken chairs with peeling shellac that are scattered throughout the lab and rips open the Velcro fasteners on his reflective strips. "When we're up against the unknown, shouldn't we use every tool we have, especially our eyes?"

"Any luck?"

"Nope, and it may not pan out. This pattern reflects the model, not the raw data. The raw data just look like static, noise. Chaos."

"Maybe you're looking at the wrong variables."

"Maybe." He smiles. "Maybe we don't know what variables to look at, or maybe there are too many for us to wrap our brains around. The human brain can only handle three or four related factors at once, seven in rare cases."

"Our methods are too crude! They require huge sample sizes, and demand more data than we can collect." Connie's knee-jerk response reflects her own doubts regarding the current approach to discovering what lies behind all too many of the public health problems she and her cohorts must investigate.

"Eureka!"

"One of these days, Isaiah will say that, and it will be true," says a high, hard voice in an unfamiliar accent. Connie turns to see a tall, dark-haired man in a once white coat reaching up toward Isaiah. As the parrot's gray feet slowly release the perch and grasp his sleeve, he asks quietly, "You wanted to see me?"

"Yes, Dr. Vanier. My name is Dr. Connie Martin and I'm here from the CDC to investigate the outbreaks of birth defects—"

"Come with me," he interrupts, turning stiffly, left hand in his pocket, right hand deftly helping the bird onto his left shoulder.

Something about Dr. Vanier frightens Connie. She pauses and looks anxiously at the young man, who looks back with just a touch of concern. "Dr. Vanier is, um, works on his own a lot. He's not much used to people."

Connie follows the researcher to his inner office, where he sits behind a desk dotted with towering piles of papers and journals. As the parrot stares intently at her, Dr. Vanier takes a small amount of chewing tobacco from an open tin and puts a neat wad into his left cheek. Connie seats herself in an oaken chair that reminds her of the time she was called to the principal's office in the fourth grade.

Doing her best to ignore the parrot, and Dr. Vanier's tonguing and chewing of tobacco, Connie explains the reason for her visit. "I have some samples for you. We were up at Leadville today to see the case mothers, and we happened on some green surface water behind the town—"

"Your stature. What's the explanation?"

Connie tips her head forward and looks at Dr. Vanier from under her eyebrows—her true predatory eye—and hisses, "Your accent. What's the explanation?"

"I was born in Lichtenstein, and studied in Leiden. But as you can tell, I have nearly lost my accent."

Connie sits dead still for a minute and then leans back in her chair. This man, ostensibly a scientist, believes and says what he pleases. Wondering whether Ira recommended the consult as a malicious joke, her mind runs over what it would take to find another scientist who knows the Colorado environment, and who understands its potential effects on human health. That would definitely create a delay, and might even fail. "There is nothing wrong with being short," she replies coldly, for the thousandth time.

"Yes, but you are abnormally short."

"I am unusually short."

"Yes, but in your field, what is unusual is abnormal, is it not?"

"Not necessarily. A feature that's statistically unusual may be clinically normal."

He laughs derisively. Pulling his left hand out of his pocket, he holds it up to show reduced fourth and fifth digits with only one joint each. "Well, doctor, what would you say to this? Abnormal or unusual?"

Connie feels a stirring of compassion. His anomaly is trivial, but unusual enough to cause many people to withdraw into pity or cruelty. "In isolation, it's a minor anomaly of no clinical significance. As you know, everyone has two or three such dysmorphic features, whether seen or not."

"Abnormal or unusual?"

"Abnormal in the sense that everyone has abnormalities."

"Is it Turner syndrome?"

Connie presses her elbows into her sides. "My mother was short. That's all."

"Eureka!"

"Ah," he says, as if about to corner her. "And what was her ancestry?"

"You'd rather turn the tables on me than help me help those children?"

"You interest me. That's all."

"What are you, a geneticist?"

"I have studied many disciplines. You may think of me as a medical anthropologist."

"My mother was born in Bolivia."

"Ah, Indian blood," he says with a deep breath of satisfaction. "Why do you hide it? Are you ashamed?"

"I'm proud of my mother! My family is my business, that's all!"

"Not quite all, I think. Your height is a part of your family legacy, and the key to many important theories. Are you aware of mitochondrial inheritance?"

"Of course I am! Mitochondrial DNA passes from mother to child in the cytoplasm of the egg. The father contributes nothing to mitochondrial inheritance."

"Eureka!"

Dr. Vanier spits his tobacco into a hidden wastebasket and leans back, pressing his fingertips together. "We carry within us the coded stories of all who came before. When the Conquistadors took Indian wives, they peopled the Americas with the likes of you. Your body tells a story that children study in school, but don't notice in life."

His dissatisfied look reappears. "You should be fat! Are you diabetic?"

"I don't have time to eat!" Connie stands and leans on his desk, hands spread, her eyes on his. "I spend too much time with people who feel too sorry for themselves to help people with real problems!"

Dr. Vanier raises his eyebrows as if giving leisurely consideration to a casual remark. "I can't help them by doing unnecessary assays."

"What do you mean, unnecessary?"

"Please, sit down. Make yourself comfortable. We've already done an extensive environmental risk assessment in Leadville. We scientifically sampled the soil, if you can call it that, the surface water, and the ground water, and then analyzed all of the samples for heavy metals and other potentially hazardous components. We found very high levels of lead, but it was not biologically available."

"What do you mean, not biologically available?"

"I mean that the lead was elemental, the kind that goes straight through the digestive tract without being absorbed."

Connie stares at him, and then at the bird, which leans toward his master's head protectively. Dr. Vanier may be odd, but she can't believe he would make up a story that could disgrace him if contradicted by any of his many colleagues in the area. She sits down on the edge of her chair. "I see. And do you suspect any environmental factor in connection with these clusters?"

Dr. Vanier raises his palms and his eyebrows. Connie nods blankly, hoists her bag back onto her shoulder, and heads for the doorway feeling the same way she did when leaving the office of an old dentist who didn't believe in numbing medicine.

As she puts one wobbly foot out into the neutral zone of the hallway, another, much larger foot comes in from the other direction. Suddenly, Connie is sitting on the ground, staring up at a stocky older man whose expression of kindly sorrow seems at odds with his leonine gray mane and beard, yellow teeth, and large brown eyes. He sighs and, without saying anything, extends his hand to lift her gently from the floor. As they silently pick up her scattered items, and Connie recovers from the shock of the fall, she feels comforted by the man's stolid solidity.

Handing her the last stray pen, his eyes express recognition as he asks, "Are you the doctor from the Centers for Disease Control?"

Connie nods in astonishment.

"I asked Dr. Weinstein to let me know when you arrived. I wanted to show you something."

The fact that Weinstein didn't mention this piques her interest. "What?"

"Come with me."

The leonine man leads her back into the suite and on into a connecting office, studiously ignoring Vanier and the parrot. The tiny office contains four of the latest computer workstations, several office chairs, a desk, and several large filing cabinets. From the framed certificates on the wall, and the mail lying next to the nearest computer keyboard, Connie deduces that the gray-maned man, William Whitburn, is a chemist and Professor of Environmental Studies.

Professor Whitburn switches on the computer monitor, and begins telling Connie the reasons for his interest in her investigation: He is working with a division of the Health Department that is fighting with Weinstein over turf and resources. It's a story she has heard too many times, in too many contexts. It doesn't hold her interest. As she watches the computer screen blink on, she wills a light to turn on in her mind.

"Here, you see? This is it!" William Whitburn's proclamation is accompanied by a lovely smile that raises her skepticism. She wouldn't be surprised if he claimed to be showing her the colors of her angel.

Connie looks at the screen, with her first impression being that it is very pretty. The graphic image, which resembles the isobars of a topographical map with fiery, soft-edged peaks of color in a sea of blue and green, shifts as Professor Whitburn's gnarled fingers clickety-clack at his keyboard. Unimpressed, and unsure of what she is looking at, she raises her eyebrows. "See what?"

His voice is patient and kindly, and she feels a sudden wish that he was her father, and didn't have to work closely with the bitter Vanier and the petty politicians at the Health Department.

"This is based on a prototype of a geographic information system the Colorado School of Mines is using to combine data from the Bureau of Land Management and other agencies. This is the graphic image we see when we correlate mineral deposits with the locations of your cases. The red areas indicate case hot spots."

"Let me guess. You ran hundreds of variables."

"Yes."

"And had no a priori hypotheses, just spatial correlations."

"Yes. It's hypothesis-generating research. But as you can see, the cases aren't random with regard to every parameter. Those parameters could be clues."

"Or they could be chance findings. Coincidences."

"We can't prove anything statistically, of course, but we can discover clues with our eyes, see patterns that we can't perceive any other way. We can use what we find to develop hypotheses."

"This is qualitative, not quantitative research."

"Yes, exactly. Empirical best guesses unaffected by noise, or scatter or ignorance or preconceived notions."

"Is that what the fellow outside your office is working on?"

"Yes."

"I don't know what to think." Connie lets out a sigh and plops into a soft-seated chair next to Whitburn. The seat lets out a whoopee-cushion noise, but Connie doesn't feel ridiculous or angry—she feels safe. She once felt this way around Dr. Cowan, but has learned that his eyes are always turned upward; he is not his own man. He is the chattel of political appointees, and always limits his thinking accordingly—which saves his subordinates from having to do so.

Connie can spot a fatherless child at fifty paces—they are mirrors that reflect weaknesses she does not want to see, with souls open to her as if they are fellow members of a gang that cannot be escaped. Able to see the void where fathering should have been, she can also sometimes guess the reason for it. The tense ones tend to have fathers blinded by alcohol or discontent, ambition or ignorance; the helpless ones may have fathers disappointed by their own elusive fathers; and the abjectly angry are apt to have fathers like hers, who were missing from the start.

But she sometimes misses this in children who are ready for a father who will fill the blank with love; in adults who have entered a patriarchal calling like medicine, science, or the church; or when the father state has protected its damaged children from uncaring, worldly chaos. And although medicine has provided this for her, she is always drawn to the father she never had.

She'd like to ask Whitburn to advise her, but there is already a father figure on this investigation. Sighing wistfully, Connie's predatory gaze relaxes into a soft appeal. "How do we keep from drowning in data? Information can reveal true patterns, and also false ones. I'm sure you know that if you have enough data, you will see many patterns that reflect layers and layers of causes and correlates. We rely on the premise that our theories bypass all those variables. We assume that we can do better than chance."

"What is statistics but a way of predicting what we don't understand?"

"But what is the significance of any statistical association if it lacks meaning?"

"Our eyes can perceive more than our rational minds."

"And more—and less—than is real."

Connie watches the monitor as Professor Whitburn clacks the keys. One after the other different patterns emerge, some quite colorful, some even beautiful. They remind Connie of the old fluoroscopic studies and the new, ever-finer CT scan images. They are hypnotic, siren images that fool almost everyone into believing that when they see more, they see what matters.

Connie knows better. She has studied medical decision making as part of her training. She knows from signal detection theory that the desire to see something in an x-ray leads to over-detection in the same way that reluctance leads to under-detection. She knows that no test is perfect, not even a laboratory test performed to atomic precision by million-dollar machines wearing the technological cloaks of modern wizardry. She also knows that tests are no better than the intentions, perceptions, concepts, and skills of the people who use them.

"Our eyes see what we expect," she counters. "We make of it what we want to."

"What is the point of being objective when we have no clues at all?"

"Do these red blobs correspond to metals? Anything that could relate to bone, for example?"

"This one is selenium," Whitburn points out.

"A trace mineral essential to health."

"But poisonous in large quantities."

"How would this get into pregnant women? Is it in the drinking water?"

Professor Whitburn goes to the filing cabinet and wrestles with a several-pound stack of accordion folded, perforated computer paper in the hanging files. "We didn't see it in the drinking water database. And the Health Department found nothing in their investigations of mine run-off."

"What do your colleagues think of your work?"

Whitburn looks at the connecting door to Vanier's office as if to gently chastise it. "They don't like it. It doesn't fit in with their ideas."

"Good. That means you're on to something new. That's what we need."

As Whitburn smiles, Connie has the strange notion that he is purring, but the noise is coming from the computer.

"Look, this method looks really promising, a great tool for the future," she tells him. "But right now, our outbreak investigation and your research are like two dots with fifteen, thirty, or a hundred missing dots in between." Connie opens her purse and retrieves a card from its depths. "If you figure out how to turn this virtual tea leaf display into a viable theory, call me. Please."

Professor Whitburn holds up the card with a nearly impassive expression in which Connie can read disappointment.

"I don't want to be the detective who lifts every fingerprint in the busy bar. We have no kind of case to guide us at this point. I can't afford to do it anyway; my budget is tiny. We can come out and look around, and that's about it. But you're here, and you have tenure. Am I right?"

The professor nods dolefully, despite his gray mane reminding Connie of a disappointed puppy.

"You're the one who can and should run with this. If we get better data on the cases, I'll be happy to share it—and control data from Atlanta or local birth records, without identifiers of course."

With this, Professor Whitburn smiles again. Connie is pleased that he is pleased, and sees that this offer is, perhaps, what he wanted all along. She stands in the warm glow of accord and shakes his hand. Then, threading through the maze of halls leading to the lobby, where she will call a cab, she gets lost in the labyrinth of her mind.

The explanation for the outbreak has slipped through her fingers, as usual, like the trout she once caught with her bare hands that wriggled free and disappeared beneath the glinting surface of the water into the camouflaged streambed. Their superficial evaluation of the montane milieu yielded too little data; Professor Whitburn's method yielded too much. The pattern that she is looking for, that interlacing sequence of events in time linking insult to damage, remains hidden. They have yet to discover the tools that could solve this puzzle posed by God, which is pushing them to delve more deeply into mystery.

These thoughts shoo away the precious sense of safety and wellbeing that she felt near Professor Whitburn. The cup of her heart goes dry. She wants to call Pippie, just to hear his voice, but doesn't trust herself to talk for long, and so contents herself with thinking of him.

By the time she emerges from the taxi, and from daydreams of her darling, she is ready to gird herself and continue on her quest. She will cheer herself up with a hot chocolate mix that she picked up during an investigation in Oaxaca, and which she always brings with her—a mix of baking cocoa, cinnamon, sugar, and cayenne that she can make with any hotel hot pot.

Sipping her special beverage, Connie feels strong enough to commune with her thoughts before dialing in and trading reports with her man-child, Ramón; and her bastard half-brother in the cause, that feet-of-clay pile of semi-sentient *adama,* Weinstein— who she will take to task as part of her mission to do her level best by all children whose fathers have failed to protect them.

Still in the thrall of her father wish, she puts off the calls, deciding instead to take a shower with the hope that it will steel her resolve. She talks herself up, ignoring her belly as she reminds herself of her vocation. Others may take creation for granted: They may keep to the animal realm of slothful ignorance, or pillage their natural mother like parasitic children who leave her no recourse but the grave. Connie will not do these things.

Comforting herself with soaps and lotions and scents that remind her of flowers, Connie renews her oath to protect her patients, private and public. She resolves, again, that she will not abandon any two-legged bit of clay to sloth or ignorance, as if it was an animal destined to be unaware of its genesis. Then she rededicates her energy and creativity to the sheltering care of those whose hearts, faces, or spirits have empty places revealing the neglect of gods—and fathers—who abandoned them in their hour of need.

5

Errors

✝

Connie watches little William Kovolitz breathe as he sleeps in his incubator in the glass-walled infant ward at Children's Hospital, irritated at having wasted time on a false lead, a case with no midline defect of any kind. Earlier, when she called to pick up her messages, Dr. Weinstein's secretary gave her baby William's name as the most recent case reported from Alamosa, then added that he had been admitted to Denver Children's Hospital for surgery. Partly to avoid a trip to Alamosa, Connie rushed over to examine the baby, who had an isolated cleft lip just like his father's. Fortunately, she was able to reassure the parents that the baby was not part of the cluster, and to share the relief they felt when they left with their over-tired three-year-old. Making a mental note to review Ramón's methods for case verification, Connie gathers up her things to leave.

Taking a last look at the clean but blank yellow walls and the infants crying in their separate, blue-sheeted enclosures, she feels suddenly isolated, and the idea of returning to her all-beige hotel room to be alone with doubt and worry makes her claustrophobic. But the thought of walking the streets to get the feel of the town and the people, as she often does when traveling, does nothing to relieve the feeling. She wants desperately to talk with someone, preferably a friend and confidante like Melissa, with whom she has been in touch less and less frequently since they went on to separate careers, but for whom she still feels a strong affinity.

Connie considers visiting Melissa, whom she knows would be able to provide solace. They could renew their friendship, and since Melissa has always been a good cook, they could also have an excellent meal. Buoyed by this time-efficient and productive plan, Connie threads her way through the crowded hallway to the pay phone beyond the nurse's station and dials the number on Melissa's card. When Dan answers, he sounds unfriendly, but he relays the message that Melissa wants Connie to come to dinner, and invites her to come by at seven.

Connie hangs up elated, but soon realizes that she still faces a stretch of idle solitude. To crush her desperation, she decides to fill up the time by editing a report, and by meeting the elusive Dr. Kazanjian. He has not yet written a pre-surgical note in baby William's chart, and should therefore be coming by before he leaves for the day.

Connie goes back to sit in the chair by the baby's crib, then takes out a copy of the report of her team's investigation of a cluster of ventricular septal defects in Tonga. When she finishes marking her edits, an hour has passed, and Dr. Kazanjian still has not arrived. Restless and impatient, Connie watches from the door until she sees a tall man with coal black hair and graying temples enter and approach the counter of the nurse's station. He banters with a blushing nurse while deftly clipping a page into a medical chart. His starched white coat and confident, precise air perfectly fulfill the stereotype of a successful surgeon. When he looks up, she recognizes his face from a photo in the lobby.

Connie goes ahead of him to baby William's crib and waits for Kazanjian. An officious nurse in yellow scrubs comes by to take the baby's vital signs, after which a grandmotherly volunteer with a tight, gray bun and large brooch comes to feed him.

After a few minutes, Connie looks out at the nurse's station again and sees that it is deserted. She stops, blocking the doorway in her confusion. She had been certain that Dr. Kazanjian would come to see little William, but she must have made some kind of mistake. Perhaps the man she saw was someone else, or perhaps he had examined the baby earlier in the day, and returned only long enough to put his note in the chart.

Even so, Connie is convinced that she had seen him at the nurse's station; and the family did tell her they had not yet met him. Perhaps he had examined the baby while she was on the phone? How foolish of her to have missed that! Frustrated, she walks to the nurse's station and takes down the Kovolitz chart, which falls open to an elegant note from Dr. Kazanjian. Word-processed and printed out, it is impressive—complete, articulate, precise, and nuanced, not to mention free of typos and stray marks. She reads the whole note, from the chief complaint to the plan, which reads smoothly, yet makes no more sense to her than a string of random letters and numbers created by a foreigner who would see the text as visual rather than logical.

Connie stares absently at the multicolored forms and disposable supplies arrayed in niches above the nurse's desk, recalling in a blur a hundred midnights when she wrote notes while on call. She squeezes her eyes shut until she sees bright white lights, and tells herself that she is getting rusty from too much deskwork, or losing her mental acuity from being pregnant. Walking slowly back to the Kovolitz crib, she asks whether the nurse or volunteer had seen Dr. Kazanjian. They had not, nor had any of the other staff.

Racing back to the counter, she pauses to rest her hand on the bracingly cold, rounded edge of stainless steel, then sits down to reread the note. It makes a certain kind of sense: It would please the most demanding administrators, insurance agents, regulators, and defense lawyers for whom information is laboriously produced and stored.

The only problem is, this note has *nothing* to do with the patient. The name and identifying data correspond to baby William, but the findings of the physical exam are perfectly detailed records of the the findings she saw that very morning in baby Hector up in Leadville—from the deep, midline facial cleft to the missing ears.

The data in baby William's chart are perfect. And perfectly false.

6

Advice

✝

"Having any trouble with the altitude?"

"No. No problem. Other than nosebleeds. The dry air makes a big change from Atlanta."

"Altitude sickness can be unpredictable," Melissa says dubiously.

For the last hour, Connie has been trying to talk with Melissa at the picnic table in the back yard, but every sentence has been cut short by Dan, who seems to be sniping at Melissa in a dogged bid for Connie's full attention.

At least they are in the last leg of the long flight of this meal, which was preceded by an unpleasant wait at the barbecue during which Dan updated her on his life with a list of covert complaints and ugly Freudian displacements that put Connie squarely in the middle of his marital discord. All the while, she has been feeling something unpleasant that she cannot quite pinpoint, which she now realizes is disgust. Dan is not the friend he had been during their first year of medical school, when he was independent— fiercely so—and ready to stand against the tide of harm that threatened to engulf his most vulnerable patients, inside and out.

At that time, when death in all its insidious forms failed to faze him, she had been proud to introduce him to Melissa. Happy when Dan took Missy into the wilderness that mended her deep Scandinavian brooding and her fresh heartbreak.

But now he is a whiner, ready to draw persecution, ready to stab his loved ones in the back—or from any direction that accident or calculation opens to the knife of his thieving need for self-approval at all costs. He has cached his old self so far from sight that he could be taken for a hollow man.

"Melissa says you're working at a doc-in-the-box. How do you like it?"

"You won't find me wussing out."

"So you don't like it."

"While you're jetting around the world, I see the same things over and over again. No prevention, no continuity, no community, no progress."

"Why do it then?

His bitter contempt hangs in the air like a cloud of defoliant. "I want to help the needy."

"You don't sound like you mean that."

"I'm holding my finger in a dike. It's pointless, and tedious."

"You want the dike to burst?"

"I want the social services net to do its job. If our patients got services when they needed them, they wouldn't show up in my examining room after it's too late."

Dan frowns and shrugs. A moment ago, he was full of angry contempt; now he is wounded and offended.

"Are you getting up into the mountains enough?"

That question brings out a better side of Dan, who is happy to take off on a tangent about fly fishing, which leads into another about backcountry skiing. As he tells the story of last weekend's drive to Red Rocks, his enthusiasm returns, and she breathes more easily. While he talks, she assumes her predatory look, thinking of other doctor marriages that she has known, and of her notion that their misery is what comes of competition.

This, however, is something else. When Dan goes in to retrieve a serving plate, Connie sits next to Melissa and whispers, "What happened to him?"

Melissa sighs. "He feels that the AMA has turned doctors into employees, and then into technology managers managed by technologies that have more to do with the economy than with medicine."

"Progress comes at a price."

"So does the illusion of control. You and I know that things aren't what they seem to be when we're in the clinic processing patients as fast as we can."

"Ugh."

"Yeah. Ugh." Melissa takes a gulp of iced tea. "Plus, he's really envious of your success—and intimidated by you."

"Me? That's pathetic. I'm a budget-less peon."

"Not so much. Medicine's in a bad way. People are exiting early."

Connie feels a burst of anger that threatens to become a missile of sorrow. She wipes away a tear that she hopes Melissa does not see.

But Melissa says softly, "Look, Connie, I'd like to think you're deeply moved to see me, but I've never seen you like this, not even when your first patient died. Is there something you want to tell me?"

Connie bursts into tears. The noise from her nose sounds like a water fountain spurting before it flows; she pulls a paper napkin from a box on the picnic table and honks into it.

"As soon as we eat, let's get out of here. I need your advice."

"Sure. You and I can go to my office and then … you can visit with Dan afterward. Okay?"

After they have finished eating, and Dan has accepted that

Connie has work to do and needs Melissa's help, he goes to cycle in City Park as the two friends drive off in the direction of her office. But before they have gone a block, Connie says "Let's take a walk."

"Yes, let's!"

Melissa heads for Cheesman Park, and soon they are enjoying a walk on its circumferential path.

"Let's talk politics first," Connie says.

"Politics?"

"Tell me what you know about Colorado Parents for Healthy Babies."

"Oh. Well, CPHB is about ten moms with a lot of supporters in certain areas, especially up in Leadville. They've got the ear of a state senator who's been pressuring the Health Department on their behalf."

"The group's name makes it sound broader," Connie says in a disappointed tone.

"I wish! Parents of sick kids always band together around a diagnosis or a disability. They don't see the big picture. Keeps their lives simple, I suppose."

"So, the group has only a few supporters?"

"I wouldn't say that. They have a huge amount of popular support right now. Every pregnant woman in the state thinks she's at risk."

"So they have the false sense of sharing a problem."

"What do you mean, false?" Melissa asks.

"I mean if there is an outbreak, and I'm not sure there is, facial cleft may be only one of many outcomes, the one that gets noticed because it's the most damaging and distressing."

"What do you mean?"

"I mean we always focus on one diagnosis, but that's probably a mistake. While it's right for treatment, it may be wrong for outbreak investigations."

"I still don't follow."

"If there's an environmental insult, the consequences probably depend on things like week of gestation, the mother's metabolism, and countless cofactors."

"So, you're saying that women exposed to a toxin might deliver babies with a whole range of problems?"

"Or not deliver them at all."

"I see. You're not sure how to define cases, so you go with the obvious."

"Exactly."

"At least you have a place to start."

"I don't know if we do. That's why I need your help. Can you come to the hospital with me now?"

"My goodness. This is serious, then."

"Yes. I want your opinion on a case."

"Sure, if it would help. But Connie, is that all? You said let's talk politics first. What's second?"

"Let's talk in the car."

"How very mysterious." Once they are rolling through the darkening streets, Melissa demands an answer. "So, what's bugging you?"

Connie sucks in her breath and holds it. She is no longer in the mood to tell Melissa anything, but her feelings are like lava that's about to erupt—she can't ignore the situation much longer, Finally, she rattles the knob of the window handle and mutters, "I'm pregnant."

"Oh, my!" Melissa turns onto a busy street. "Congratulations! But you don't sound happy. Are you worried about your job? Oh, of course! You're worried about birth defects!"

"Yes, but it isn't that." Connie speaks softly as her chin sinks into her chest.

Melissa checks her rearview mirrors, moves over two lanes and pulls up to the curb, tires squealing. Connie feels like she is riding in a formula one car that is making a pit stop. "Are you—Pea, you're not thinking about abortion? You've always been against it!"

"I've always been against pregnancy, and so has Pippie! How could I be a mom, and how could he be a dad? He plays computer games all day!"

"Is that what he said?"

"I—" Connie tries to think of an excuse, but she knows that any will sound ridiculous if she says it out loud. "I haven't told him."

Melissa's mouth opens. She stares at Connie, pauses, and then finally speaks.

"Pea, you have to tell him, and then give him time to react and adjust and work out what he feels and thinks. Most men live in denial. They don't want kids until they see their own, and then they do."

Connie grips the car seat as if she is worried it will leave without her. "What if Pippie leaves me?"

"You mean the way your dad left your mom?"

Connie shakes her head. "A lot of men want sex without consequences."

"Your mom wanted the consequences."

"She handled her situation. I have to handle mine."

"Have you talked to your mom? She's from around here, isn't she?"

"Don't breathe a word to anyone about that!"

"But why, Pea? Your job might be easier if people knew you

were from this area."

"If Weinstein finds out I'm Hispanic, he'll send me out schmoozing. I'll never get on with the investigation!"

Melissa's face settles into the clinical mask she uses to say things like, *How long were you on the alien mother ship?*

"You're Hispanic?"

"Yes."

"You told me you were Mormon."

"Did I?"

"You said your father was the smallest man on Samoa."

Connie laughs. "What a story."

"Pea, what's going on here?"

"It's no one's business."

"Don't try to weasel out of this. You've been lying to me for years. Why would you do that?"

Connie hadn't thought of it that way. She was a child of poverty storing her few secrets in a box. She contained them by sealing and burying them so that others could not release their carefully contained poisons.

"Have you ever seen me betray a confidence?" Melissa asks quietly.

Connie shakes her head. She knows that Melissa doesn't want to do harm, but Connie can't trust her to recognize the harm in stigma that only those marked can understand.

"Why would you abuse my trust that way?" Melissa protests.

Suddenly tired of the lies, Connie realizes she has long since lost track of them all. They are like burdens that she has bundled and carried on her shoulder for years, until she can barely remember how it might feel to release their weight. "You would never understand."

"The only way you can be sure I wouldn't, is if you try me and I don't."

At this point, Connie feels ready to take down one of the burdens. *One at a time.* "The reason I'm small and dark is my mother is a refugee from Bolivia. A powerful neighbor took her land and killed most of her family. A church here in the San Luis Valley helped her to escape and gave her sanctuary."

Melissa is frowning. She can't see a reason for hiding this.

"You probably think Hispanics and Latinos are all the same, but they're not. Hispanics in the Valley have roots going back to the conquistadors. They don't accept Mexicans, and they never accepted us. My friends were all Mormons."

"So, you were Hispanic, and you were excluded by Hispanics?"

"My mother spoke Quechua and Spanish, and practiced both religions. We didn't know anyone else who did."

Melissa continues to frown.

"For God's sake don't tell anyone! The Church accepted us as Catholic. If they knew—!"

"So the Church wouldn't like that?"

"No! They used to kill people who kept the old faiths alive!"

"They don't do that anymore, Connie, if only because they can't."

"Melissa, I want to feel safe!"

Connie shivers. Melissa's eyes are like security cameras collecting evidence that will expose Connie to the judgment and condemnation of the world; she cannot bear to look. Her mind has ugly names for the weakness that led her to speak so openly to this friend, who might at any moment turn on her with the violence of hatred or evangelism.

Connie adds in a whisper, "I pray every day that no one recognizes me!"

"I will not breathe a word to anyone about any of this if that's your heart's desire, but think about it. You may be safer than you know."

"Promise you won't tell anyone!" Connie insists.

"I promise."

Connie takes a deep breath.

"And your father?" Melissa asks.

"I'm not ready to talk about that!"

"Okay. Okay!"

Melissa pulls away from the curb and drives in silence like a chauffeur who is not allowed opinions about her employer. After entering the cramped parking lot of Children's Hospital, she swings into a deserted space.

Connie wipes her face again. "Before we get out, give me your advice about what to do."

"I did, Pea. Look at everything you are, including your profession. The new life in you depends on you, and you were born to care for it. It's what you are, what you do. You'll never forgive yourself if you let fear lead you to abort the flesh of your flesh and Pip's flesh.

"What if the baby has a problem surgery can't fix! Think of the suffering. First do no harm. Remember?"

"If you discover a problem, you'll figure out what to do, as always."

"But how can I do what I do if I let this happen?"

Melissa unclicks her seat belt and reaches over to give her friend an awkward, sideways hug. "Think about our whole conversation, and then tell me what you think."

"I'm damned if I do and damned if I don't!"

"Have you considered the possibility that this is good news, but you can't see it because you had a rough childhood and you've seen too many funny-looking kids? Kids teach you to be a mother. You don't need to know everything right now. Think of your marriage, and the way you learn as you go."

"I never want to end up like my mom, abandoned and unemployed and responsible for a baby no one wants!"

"Oh, Connie. You're none of those things! Give your mom some credit. You turned out great!"

"I have to—I have to deal with these things in my own way."

"By all means. Tell me what you want me to do."

"Just help me with this investigation."

"Whatever I can, I'll do."

Melissa locks up the car and they walk toward the row of streetlights that nearly obscures the deep blue void of the sky. Connie sees the brightly lit hospital entrance ahead, and, feeling its promise of safety, wants to run toward it and into it.

But Melissa deliberately slows her pace, processing things as they make their way across the street to the hospital.

Connie's anger dissipates like steam from a teakettle that has been removed from the stove. She is, above all, alone and afraid. Her anger turns inward, and she feels a cold well of guilty fear. Melissa is a lifeline, the only friend on whom she can possibly rely. If Melissa does not want to help, Connie will have no one, and she decides—without realizing it—to test the loyalty of her old friend by raising the fraught issue of religion that is one of the barriers between the atheist, secular, Jewish Dan and the spiritual but not-religious Melissa.

Connie blurts, "I should go to confession!" then watches Melissa's face for any sign of partiality, any impulse to annihilate Connie's reality. She sees nothing, and Melissa says nothing.

"Well? What do you think of what I just said?"

"If you want to go to confession, you should go. Do you

want me to help you find a church in town? I could ask around."

Connie's heart constricts around regret. The disloyalty is hers, and hers alone. "There's a little parish church near my hotel. I keep passing it. I can't stop thinking about it. But I'm too angry to go in, and too afraid."

"Do you want me to go with you?"

"No, no, no!"

"Okay, okay. I'm just trying to help."

Connie tries to calm herself. *One thing at a time.* Her awareness becomes still enough to see that her God-sense is running through her brain like a naked woman searching for shelter in a damp thicket: At every turn, it hopes to discover refuge but finds only thorny complexity. Connie is desperate to reduce the overwhelming detail of life to a pattern like a garden of earthly delight, but it is a stubborn wilderness of tangled branches that form disparate, fragmented realities.

Connie becomes aware that they have crossed the cold dark street and have nearly reached the sacred place that she knows best, the place where science offers what healing it can—through her, and through Melissa and Dan and all their colleagues. It is the place she can trust because she has it in her power to distinguish fakery from grace, and because she and they have vowed to do everything in their power to make it safe for all.

As they are about to enter, Connie feels Melissa's hand on her upper arm. "I do have one last bit of advice, which is to think about what secrets do."

"I know what they do. They protect people!"

"What they really do is spread fear," Melissa counters.

"How can you say that?"

"Think of what it would be like to reveal your secrets. Not to regurgitate them undigested, just to tell the story of your life for little girls like you who think they're alone in the world with a big problem. Consider what it would be like for you to be open; and then, if you want to, try it. In the meantime, if you're going to hide your roots, hide them well. If people find out you're hiding your past, they'll think you're ashamed of being a local, or of being Hispanic, or of your indigenous roots. They'll take it personally, and you'll deprive them of the chance to be on your side, and to take heart from your struggles."

Not on your life. "Okay, I'll think about it. If you think about your marriage. Dan's awful these days. You should think about leaving him."

"The problem is that I don't do enough. Dan does far more than his share."

"Of taking care of his car, and his house, and his other possessions?"

"We have active problems. We have to work on them," Melissa says half-heartedly.

"Don't kid yourself, Melissa. He's angry, which is making him mean, demanding, and narcissistic. You will never be able to do enough to satisfy him, and he won't either. He's weak, and he'll weaken you too, if you let him."

"Isn't it interesting how easily we see the problems of others," Melissa says with a rueful laugh.

"And fortunate. Dan thinks, or, rather, his adaptive unconscious is programmed to assume, that he should enforce what he thinks is exemplary self-discipline or self-denial, but he's just hurting himself by running from his weakness instead of facing it."

"Thank you for that helpful consult, which I didn't ask for, in case you didn't notice."

"Just doing you a favor."

"Fair enough," Melissa says with a sad smile.

Inside the empty, darkened hall, Connie looks around as if she is afraid of being overheard. She pulls Melissa to the side, near the wall, as if it is more private, and whispers in her friend's ear, "I'll show you a couple of things and then we'll talk somewhere private. Okay?"

"More secrets?"

Connie's irritation sparks like static electricity. She hurls a verbal sideswipe. "Your eyes are getting puffy. In med school they only got puffy if you'd been up all night."

"Gee, thanks." Melissa laughs incredulously, recovering her patient love of her dear friend, one of only a handful of people in the world to whom Melissa would entrust her life.

As Connie sighs and disappears around the corner into a maze of corridors, Melissa dashes after her, dodging a gantlet of slow-moving families trailed by grandparents and toddlers. Finally, arriving breathless at the bedside of baby William Kovolitz, who is lying like an upside-down beetle between the anxious faces of his parents, they witness his agitated sister acting out the family tension by biting her father's arm.

Connie introduces herself and Melissa, after which Melissa does a cursory examination of baby William. They take their grave faces out of the room and down the busy hallway to the nurse's station, where Melissa reads the note in the chart and sighs deeply. "Okay, it's all very clear. I understand your concern. Let's go somewhere and talk in private."

As they exit the front door of the hospital, Connie grabs Melissa's arm again and hisses in her ear. "Can you believe it? He put a fake note in the chart! He put it in without examining the patient at all, which means that he's going to operate on a kid he's never seen! He may even have created this cluster just to bring money into the hospital, or his own pockets! We have to stop him!"

"Shush! Let me think. I'm going to need a margarita."

"I can't have a drink in my condition!"

"Have a steamed milk, then."

Melissa says nothing while she drives, but expressions flicker across her face like weather systems over a mountain peak—dark and sunny, stormy and then dark again. Connie keeps quiet with difficulty until her thoughts wander into a dark forest of past sorrows. Finally, Melissa parks, and they enter a corner restaurant with a dark, wood-paneled interior and cool, stale air that smells of fried fish. The lighting inside is so low that Connie sees only rows of high-backed booths and a mirrored wall lined with glass shelves holding colorful spirits and mixers.

They wait several minutes to be seated, during which time Melissa is pensive and Connie lapses into a state of alert fatigue that promises a wakeful night. When they are seated, and Melissa has ordered a margarita and Connie an herbal tea, Melissa says, "I know him, you know, not personally, just as a colleague. He's operated on a couple of my kids. He's got magic hands. But there have been whispers."

"Whispers?"

Melissa leans forward and speaks quietly. "You know how guys like him walk a fine line between being confident enough to deliver the impossible, and arrogant enough to believe they're above all the rules? Rumor has it he's crossed that line."

"Melissa! Out with it! This is no time to worry about being a gossip!"

"This is exactly the time to worry! He's left himself wide open. If we don't handle this well, he could lose his confidence—and his license. My patients need him."

Connie folds her arms and glares. "He's about to operate on a baby sight unseen!"

"I get it. He's lost in virtual reality. He believes what's in the computer even as he takes liberties with what he puts into it. The point is, we shouldn't ruin him just because he's a megalomaniac who snubs the rules! We can't act out of envy. A lot of people resent his women and his sports cars and his house in Aspen and his condo in Hawaii. We have to see past all that."

"His note is a fake!" Connie exclaims, showering tiny droplets that bead up on the shiny table and glisten in the candlelight. "It's unforgivable!"

"The patient will be fine. The anesthesiologist will check the pre-ops, and in the morning, when K sees the cleft, he'll repair it perfectly. That's what matters."

"Frightening people matters too. Corruption matters."

"Let's not get caught up in the whole rock star thing. Surgeons attract everyone's attention, but the medical reality is that their patients don't walk in off the street; they come in via primary care docs. The problem isn't here in Denver. It's out there, in the mountains."

"I need to talk to people and find out what's going on. You're not enough," Connie counters in frustration.

"Of course I'm not. And I will help you. So let's move on to actual gossip. Have you heard from anyone else?"

7

Father Sean Finnegan

As Father Sean makes his way from the rectory to the confessional of the diminutive Cathedral of Our Lady of Sorrows, his brooding about the new bran cereal that Mrs. Hernandez, the housekeeper, gave him that morning for breakfast causes him to miss the gorgeous tint of purple twilight above the line of peaks on the western horizon. Self-consciously repressing his worries about his bowels, he smooths the creases between his brows so as not to frighten Mrs. Marino, who just last week complained about his glowering to Bishop Okot.

Father Sean's faith had begun as a proverbial mustard seed, flourished into a great tree, and then withered into a twisted stick. Thirty years ago, he arrived on fire to bring the Word of God to the Wild West, but lost that in his intimacy with disappointment. Denver turned out to be a self-aggrandizing cow town that had grown up along the railway and then moved to the suburbs, where it was wasting itself in a frenzy of consumption. His parish west of the downtown had been overtaken by urban decay, his pious Mexican and Italian immigrant parishioners moved away.

He is now left with a few stubborn elders and occasional floods of male illegal laborers who make more confessions of lust, battering, theft, knifing, pederasty, and murder than he can abide with hope. His forehead is creased, and his heart is grown sour with a degree of contempt for the poor that would shock

71

his childhood friends from the slums of Belfast.

Lost in thought, Father Sean halts just in time to avoid colliding with old Mrs. Benettoni, whose spine has become so bent that her nose points at her toes.

"Sure and it's a beautiful evening, Mrs. B.," he says, exaggerating the remnants of his Irish accent and turn of phrase, which comforts him while charming others. "As the Mayor might say," he adds absently. At one time he quoted the Bible, the Pope, the Bishop, and his mother, often and with precision. Over the years, however, his quotes have lost focus, finally degenerating into pleasantries in the name of any authority that comes to mind.

Giving Mrs. Benettoni's deformity a wide birth, he scuffs away along the gravel path to the sanctuary, which he finds empty, as usual, but for his clumping footfalls and the lace-clad Mrs. Marino. She is sitting in the Madonna chapel staring over a sea of votives as if willing the stone image to cry tears of blood.

Sealing himself in the confessional, he sits and fidgets briefly with his cassock, brooding about the evening news which continues to provide redundant proof that there is no God. Unable to forget the lurid pictures of listless infant bodies, their bandaged faces black and blue and helpless, he longs briefly for the solace of blame. But whom or what can he blame for this outrage against innocents? He hopes, rather than prays, that doctors and scientists will find out.

Suddenly awakening with a start, his knee bumping audibly and painfully against the wooden wall, Father Sean hears a woman's voice saying tensely, "… for I have sinned. It has been fifteen years since my last confession."

He very nearly asks why she has bothered to come at all, but clearing his throat of all that gathered there while he slept, merely inquires, "Why so long?"

"I'm only here because I'm desperate," she blurts, pausing to blow her nose.

He peers through the lattice and catches a glimpse of a well-tailored, conservative suit; an expensive overcoat; and coarse, flyaway, blue-black hair that reminds him of a young woman he once knew. He suspects that the penitent is from out of town, a guest at the new hotel two blocks away, where urban decay is giving way to urban renewal. Her energetic struggle makes him feel oddly happy. "Yes ...?" he prompts, trying not to sound too eager.

"I have committed the following sin: I have considered terminating my pregnancy!" she declares, blowing her nose again before letting loose a deep sob.

"You're not married?"

"What makes you say that?"

Father Sean fears that Mrs. Marino might hear, and after a long silence looks through the lattice again to see a face peering back at him. Startled, he looks away, but not before recognizing her from the evening news: She is the doctor who talked about the deformed babies. He is so distracted that he misses yet another part of her confession.

"... hate priests! I couldn't come back after—after what happened! He never should have done what he did! She was all by herself in a new country, and so helpless, so innocent!"

During the long silence that follows, Father Sean thinks of the babies; the penitent; and his own, long-time anger at the church, *and* at priests, whose confessions rival any for devilry. His heart is pierced with a pain so intense that he groans before gasping and falling back, then hitting his head on the wood.

Connie peers in again at the priest, for whom she feels only the most reluctant glimmer of trust, and to whom she would never have turned had she not been on the brink of a break-down. She can see graying temples, a pale, sweaty face, a panting mouth, and whitish lumps in the skin below his eyes, which she recognizes as telltale signs of high cholesterol. As she shifts in her seat, she espies plump hands that seem to be suspended above a huge belly.

Jesus Mary Joseph! She races around the crudely carved box, opens his door, and steps inside. Then, as Father Sean raises his hand as if to ward off the devil, she shakes her head, clicks her tongue, and scolds, "Look at you! You're the picture of sloth and gluttony!"

He feels her pull his arm, and then feels nothing until he wakes again, lying down surrounded by blue and red and green dots of light. He is moving. A siren blasts his ears. He must be in the back of an ambulance. Craning his neck, he sees the face of the doctor who'd been on his television, then in his confessional, and now in his ambulance. The way she looks at him, the way she is both here and not here, propels the priest into a strange state.

Everything that had been static flows; everything flat and empty turns vivid and textured and deep, as if incarnating the flow of time. A previously invisible dimension comes to life before his eyes, and he knows that he could have seen it at any time if only he had taken the trouble. The surfaces of things were always transparent in this way—or, rather, he had known that they were flimsy and facile and could be seen through.

He stares at the pregnant woman's face, behind which he sees the hand of the Divine, which is causing her to shed dark tears. Tears of blood. God lives in and behind every surface, including his own face, and has hidden from him until now in order to burn away his sins through separation. He has been purified and forgiven. *Thanks be to God! Thanks be to this dark angel, his messenger!* He weeps for joy.

When Father Sean awakens again his head is pounding, and he seems to be lying on a rock. He sees another face, one that is familiar and serene, but not angelic. It is his old friend, Brother Ben, sitting in the padded chair beside his hospital bed, snoring. He has not seen Ben since the last meeting of the Board of Trustees of his Zen Temple. Father Sean's eyelids droop. He closes them in hopes of another vision, but none comes. His heart, which must be responsible for the green light that is sweeping up and down the tiny monitor, and for the beeping noise that accompanies it, feels different to him, as if it is awake but has a hangover.

When he wakes again, he says, "Ben! Ben! Wake up."

Brother Ben Takahashi grabs the armrests of his chair and sits up abruptly, knocking his straight gray hair down over his eyes, which widen with his broad, teasing smile. "Sean! Welcome back. They had to give you a big dose of Demerol. You were overexcited. That wouldn't happen if you practiced Zazen."

"Ben, I had a vision! What you call a realization!"

"Oh. I thought you had a heart attack."

"Yes, a heart attack!" Sean laughs. "Sure and God had to attack me to give me a new heart, I was so difficult!"

"You needn't have gone to all this trouble," Ben says. "I could have told you that." He is smiling, but his eyes are somber and his crow's feet deep—a sure sign that he is distressed. He had been famously cool when he played center in Denver's Buddhist basketball league, and the largely Japanese Sensei players had jokingly talked him up as being the shortest center in the country. Now that he is a serene Zen priest, he turns to the darker emotions only on certain occasions, like illnesses and deaths and the family gatherings at which he tells stories about the internment of his parents in a nearby camp during World War II. The same war during which his uncle was killed in action, and his mother went insane.

"I want to try Zazen," Sean declares. "I'm going to listen to you from now on."

"That's too bad. I so enjoyed our arguments," Ben deadpans with a wry smile. "You'd better go to sleep. Maybe you'll wake up your old self."

"Did you see that woman who came in with me? I have to find her. I keeled over before she finished confessing. She's my Madonna—and now I have to save her baby!" Father Sean smiles and closes his eyes.

Brother Ben's eyes close too as he listens patiently to the silence beyond the beeping of the heart monitor and the dripping of the faucet in the adjacent bathroom. Although he sits up late into the night, dozing on and off, Father Sean doesn't reawaken.

When Mrs. Carmen Hernandez hears a siren come near the rectory and cut out with a little whoop, she hurries out of the rectory and approaches the flashing lights just as the ambulance rolls away. She goes directly to the sanctuary, where she comforts Mrs. Bennetoni while Mrs. Marino tells the story of Father Sean's collapse as if it had been an insult to her stern dignity. When the two women leave, Carmen lights many candles in the rack under the statue of Our Lady of Guadeloupe near the main entrance and prays for Father's healing until her bone-deep faith is fully aroused. She then recesses to the rectory, where she calls Brother Ben, Father's closest friend from his Civil Rights days. Carmen then goes to her room, which she has appointed in the way of her sister's convent room, to pray through the night, awake and asleep.

Early the next morning, Carmen gathers the paraphernalia that will make the hospital room fit for a priest, and vice-versa—including the holy oil he might need to administer the rite of extreme unction, God forbid. She then drives the old rectory rattletrap to the hospital, talks her way past a phalanx of nurses and into the cardiac care unit, and prepares the room while Brother Ben and Father Sean sleep. Then she sits in a side chair and reads his Bible while looking up now and again at the large wood and brass crucifix that she suspended from the wall-mounted television stand, where her morning telenovela is playing in silence.

Now and then, her mind wanders to her years with Father Sean. More recently, as the parish has fallen on hard times and Father Sean's spirit has ebbed, her own faith has remained as fervent and joyful as it was at her first communion, for which her mother dressed her like a princess. Having lost many things in her life, she now simply accepts the parish church and its priest the way she does the old chalice—which, although missing its jewels, still serves out the miracle of transubstantiation.

When Mrs. Hernandez crosses herself and gives thanks to God for sparing the life of Father Sean, he stirs and notices for the first time that she takes far better care of him than he deserves. She catches his eye, smiles with her brows knit, and goes to take the lid of his meal tray and to move his bedside tray to just the right spot as he pushes the button that raises the head of his bead. Leaning over his bedside tray, he inhales to draw in the aroma of chicken enchiladas past the plastic oxygen tubes in his nostrils: One side of the plate is smothered in red sauce, and the other in green sauce, just the way he likes it. Mrs. Hernandez gives an identical plate to Brother Ben, who eats from his lap in the visitor's chair, pleased that he has an excuse to pass on his wife's *saba shioyaki,* which has never been as good as his mother's.

"I see you're back to your old self," Brother Ben observes, as Father Sean wipes his chin after taking an enormous bite.

"Well, I still adore my *abuelita's* excellent enchiladas," Father Sean replies, with a nod to Mrs. Hernandez. She shakes her head at the compliment, but smooths her white hair and folds her hands over her apron to look her best as she receives the praise. "But I've had another realization, as you call it."

"You've seen your Madonna again?"

"No, no. No Madonna, no tears of blood. No, it was something else!" he replies, dropping his fork and raising both hands as if to give a benediction. Mrs. Hernandez tips her head back to look through her bifocals as she searches for traces of irony in the priest's face, but sees none. "Earlier, when I was stirring, I looked up at the image of the Son of God, wondering why he spared my life, and asking myself what I should do with the time he has given me. I started to pray—"

Father Sean was about to say "For the first time in years," but after a contrite glance at his *abuelita*—who is looking at him the way she watches the climactic scenes in *Passiones* on the Rectory television—says: "I wasn't sleeping. I couldn't have been, because I was aware of you and Mrs. Hernandez while contemplating the image of the Son. But as I prayed, a Spirit began to stir in him, and then came out of him; not in the form of a dove, but in the form of a light shaped like his image! And then he descended from the cross and walked away!"

"Mmmm," Brother Ben says skeptically. His forehead, which shows hints of doubt and worry, seems to have aged years in a day. He asks, with characteristic dry humor, "Which way did he go?"

"Well," replies Father Sean, picking up his fork with one hand and pointing through the glass wall of his room to the nurse's station with the other, "it seemed that he might go that way, but his light blended with the light in the room. I couldn't see him after that, but it wasn't because he'd gone, it was because he was everywhere, moving—flowing you might say—like the breath of life, but as light."

Hearing this, a radiance emanates from the face of Mrs. Hernandez, who crosses herself and runs out, forgetting her bag, which is typical, and the rectory dishes, which is not.

Father Sean calls after her, "Mrs. Hernandez, are you all right?" When she fails to reappear, he returns to eating his enchiladas, adding, with a full mouth, "I wonder what got into her?"

"She probably wonders what got into you. I hope she doesn't think it's a devil."

Father Sean happily returns Brother Ben's ribbing, "Oh, my friend, there is only God, there is nothing but God! I'm sure the Buddha would agree if only we could have a real conversation!"

"You can ask the Tibetans about that. They talk to the Perfect Buddha all the time."

Father Sean laughs delightedly. "Some of us need those little chats."

"You'd better have them at St. Peter's. If you have them here, the doctors might move you to the psychiatric ward."

"I'm only turning into a Holy Fool, my dear friend, and Fools can talk to as many voices as they please!"

"Is that in Leviticus? That book has some real doozies."

"Seriously, Brother Ben, I must figure out the meaning of that vision!"

When Father Sean takes the final huge bite of his enchiladas, he hears a female voice scold him sharply. "If you don't choke, you'll drown in your own blubber! You'd better pray for arthritis of the jaw!"

Brother Ben looks up at the tiny woman standing in the doorway. In the fraction of a blink, before he takes note of the color of her hair or the tension around her mouth, he senses her state of being, which is that of a cornered animal—a cat, maybe, or a fawn. Her fear evokes his compassion, and his heart goes out to her.

In the next fraction of a blink, Connie, who does not perceive Brother Ben's earthy tranquility or glowing heart, knows instantly that she likes him. "Hello, I'm Dr. Martin, just checking on the patient."

"Oh. I thought you were trying to give him another heart attack."

Father Sean swallows noisily and blurts, "I'm glad you've come. I wanted to thank you for saving my life, and to apologize for not hearing out your confession."

"So, you're the one who gave him the first heart attack!" Brother Ben interjects. "That must have been quite a confession."

"I just wanted to talk to someone. I'm not religious!"

"Are you irreligious?"

"Not exactly. It's just that I prefer science. Organized religion does a lot of harm."

"I see. When you compare the Inquisition and Hiroshima, you favor Hiroshima?"

Father Sean pulls his covers up, afraid that Connie might respond to Brother Ben's humor in the way of Bishop Okot, but she only replies in a small, raw voice, "When I look at the priests and scientists in my life, I find that the priests care for the Church, and the scientists care for the truth."

"Ah. So you like to see things exactly as they are," Brother Ben replies.

"Yes."

"Then you are a Buddhist!" he declares with a half smile. Connie laughs, and Father Sean lowers his covers tentatively, amazed that Connie appreciates Ben's sense of humor.

Brother Ben stands and gathers up the dishes and Mrs. Hernandez' bag. "I'll take these to the rectory and leave you two to do whatever it is that Catholics do when a doctor is ministering to a priest. I'm sure that's all in Leviticus as well." He pads away, waving his arm over his head as he disappears into the hallway.

"You're quite a pair!" Connie notes with a smile.

"I've lost faith in the Church from time to time, but I've never lost faith in Brother Ben, and he's never lost faith in his Zen."

Connie sits stiffly on the edge of the heavy visitor's chair and looks at Father Sean with her predatory eye. She is thinking that Denver isn't turning out as expected, and feels a pang of nostalgia for the simplicity of the cholera outbreak in Bangladesh, where everyone knew what to do and no one had had time for ambiguities or niceties—like deciding whether to treat Father Sean as a priest, or as an ordinary man.

"Would you like to make your confession now?" Father Sean asks, his brow creasing like a closing accordion. He looks at the crucifix, hoping for guidance regarding his visions and Connie's unborn child, but receives none, though he seems to hear Brother Ben advising him to meditate on his vision and to stop clinging to Connie's unborn child, which he is confusing with the Christ.

"You're on my turf now, Father. Tell me how you're feeling, and what they've told you."

"I feel fine, just a little tired. They say I may have had a heart attack and that I have to make some changes. Mrs. Hernandez will be seeing the nutritionist, and I'm going to exercise."

"Hmph. I'll have to visit you at the Rectory and make sure you follow through."

"Why don't you come for a low-fat dinner?" Father Sean offers impulsively. "You can tell me if there's anything I can do to help those poor afflicted babies."

Connie's jaw tightens, but then her eyebrows go up as she replies, "You know, Father, there is something. We have no idea what's causing this outbreak. You might be able to uncover some clues by talking to your colleagues in the mountains."

Father Sean consults the crucifix, which gives him no sign. "And what kind of clues would I be looking for?"

"Anything that might have affected the babies in utero. Any storms or spills that might affect the air or water, any new products or trends in behavior, especially any new drug use or hobby or business, people moving in or out, unusual men passing through town, flu outbreaks—anything new or different."

"That narrows it down considerably," Father Sean observes with a sly smile.

Connie forces a smile. "Thank you, Father. I'll visit tomorrow." Then she rushes out, her heels clicking like castanets.

Mrs. Hernandez has been very excited by the stream of visitors to the hospital. But when Father Sean tells her that Bishop Okot is coming to call, she is so eager to phone her friends with the news that now she must hurry to prepare for the actual event. After all, it's been years since any bishop visited her priest, and she has never even seen Bishop Okot.

The doorway suddenly fills with the tall, broad-shouldered mass of the bishop, whose mouth is turned down at the corners as if gravity might pull them into his jowls. His bulky shoulders droop at the sight of Father Sean, who represents everything that he detests about his diocese.

When Bishop Okot was elevated to the Vatican from his humble beginnings in an East African village where he had ministered to the morally lax, he felt he had arrived in the promised land, although his stay there had been brief. Despite fulfilling his duties obediently and competently, or perhaps because of it, he had been reassigned to Denver, a place where parishioners worshiped the things of this world, and the priests—especially Father Sean—were strangers to the Spirit. He would never have believed that any place could be so spiritually backward.

Father Sean reaches up to smooth out the furrows in his forehead. His shoulders sag like the Bishop's until he recalls his spiritual rebirth and exclaims eagerly, "Please, come in, come in, and tell me the meaning of my visions!"

The Bishop turns his head skeptically to one side as he steps a pace closer to Father Sean, but his shoulders rise up a notch as he asks in a deep, resonant voice, "Your visions?"

"Yes, Bishop. The first one was in the ambulance." Father Sean leans his left arm on the side rail and traces the visions in the air with his right hand, speaking first of the Madonna, and then of the Christ.

Bishop Okot takes a seat in the chair and listens attentively, his jowls and shoulders rising until he seems to float. Then, after hearing Father Sean's descriptions, smiles broadly as he provides an explanation.

"The Living Christ has come into your life at last! He has made you whole in Spirit, and the flesh will certainly follow. You will be ready to carry out your delicate assignment!"

"I don't quite follow, Bishop."

At that, the Bishop hops to his feet, motions for Mrs. Hernandez to exit, and walks lightly to the door to close it after her. Pulling the chair nearer to the hospital bed, he sits back down, elbows on the wooden arms with palms together. He speaks in a low voice, barely moving his lips or jowls as he continues, "Mrs. Marino told me about the confession you received the night you were overcome."

Father Sean puts his hand on his forehead to keep from frowning. "I can't account for it. How could she have heard it?"

"The young woman seems to have spoken loudly." The Bishop chuckles, making a sound Father Sean has never heard, and which reminds him of a bittern. "Mrs. Marino was in quite a state! She thought the young woman was accusing you!"

Father Sean stares at the green dot as it bounces along the monitor, drawing his heartbeat with increasing speed. A tiny Filipino nurse rushes in scolding, but, seeing the Bishop, crosses herself and stops abruptly. She looks at the monitor, then at the door, and admonishes in a very high-pitched voice, "Please relax now, Father. It is very important not to be excited, now. You must rest, Father, now."

"Thank you, my child." He lays obediently against the pillows and takes a deep breath. "The Bishop and I will say a prayer for relaxation."

The nurse lingers as the Bishop closes his eyes, raises his chin, and says a quiet and simple prayer. The nurse leaves, closing the door behind her with a grateful smile. Father Sean's brow grows smooth as he feels calmer.

"I have to confess, Bishop Okot, that I can't remember what happened before I passed out."

"You didn't hear the confession?"

"I don't recall it. I offered to hear it when she visited."

"You've seen her here in the hospital? That's good. I want you to see her again. I'm going to entrust you with a delicate task of importance to the Church, which won't be easy: If Mrs.

Marino is correct, the young doctor's father was a priest, and her situation was mishandled. He never acknowledged, or supported, mother or child. I want you to find him, then have him report to me his plan for taking responsibility for his error, as well as how he intends to take care of both of them."

"I see."

"By the way, your doctor says that you did not have a heart attack—so you can start today."

8

Kitchen Cabinet

On the flight to Atlanta, after the end of a distressing visit, Connie dozes and dreams, haunted by her last conversation with Melissa. The talk hadn't gone well, and it was, in retrospect, all her own fault. Melissa had been urging her to expand on the idea that Jesus' birth was part of God's plan. Connie had assumed that Melissa's aim was to get her to agree to keep the baby. Connie had snapped.

"Real marriages don't turn out according to God's plan! Look at yours! It's ugly, ugly, ugly."

Melissa had been like a woman who had just given her last dime to an old friend and was being hit up for more. She snapped, too. "Is it better to marry a man who can't leave you because he's too fat to leave the house?"

"Pippie loves me!"

"But do you love him? You don't trust him enough to tell him you're pregnant, or respect him enough to ask what he thinks and feels about it. You have a lot of work to do on your own marriage!"

Connie said sarcastically, "I'm just trying to help."

"Hating isn't helping!"

"Hating! Who's hating? I—I—this is tough love!"

"If you think your verbal abuse is love, I'd hate to be your kid," Melissa had responded.

"I'm just doing what you do!"

"Bullshit! You're the baby in every relationship you have. You don't need to figure out whether to keep the kid, you need to figure out whether to stay a kid—and you'd better do it quick. You're showing."

"I'm not showing. And I'm not abusive. I'm just telling it like it is."

"You're telling it like you see it, which means you're only seeing you. Don't try to hold a mirror up to me until you can look into it and see yourself as you are—and love what you see. When you can do that, you may be able to see me with loving eyes. Maybe."

"I do love you."

"You judge me and feel judged. The judging is all yours."

"I'm not judgmental! Dan's judgmental!"

"We've all been medically trained in the same way—trained to ignore our inner lives unless we have some religion to turn to. But you and Dan came into it from abuse and neglect. You have a great need, and no permission or opportunity to meet it. I'm probably going to convert to Judaism, or at least do the practices. What are you going to do?"

"You're the one who needs to do some kind of work on yourself. You're abusing me right now!"

"No, *you're* abusing you. You turn everything into abuse, and you project it onto everyone but yourself. Get a clue!"

Connie couldn't think of anything to say that wouldn't make Melissa seem right, and she didn't want to do that. She did not want to lose that battle, to have to accept Melissa's point of view and figure out what to do about it. *I should never have exposed myself to Melissa, or to anyone.*

"Masochism isn't a virtue, it's a vice," Melissa had continued relentlessly. "Trust me, I do see that in all of us. In Dan's anger and yours, and in my sorrow. We're all tortured by regret, and not just the big things, but every little thing, every little minute. And you're right—it's ugly, ugly, ugly."

"You're just like me, then."

"Actually, I'm not. And I'm not going to enable your abuse by accepting what you project and apologizing for it. Not anymore. I'll help your investigation as a colleague, but I won't be your friend until you want to receive and acknowledge and be grateful for what I have to give. No more pearls before swine. You decide, and let me know."

Now, on the plane, Connie realizes she's already decided. She is going to go home and tell Pippie about the pregnancy, and when she gets back to Denver she'll buy Melissa some flowers and ask her to help. She is lucky to have a friend who is so tolerant of her faults, and has never been more aware of that.

On her next trip to Denver, after Connie has apologized to Melissa and has let a few days pass, she asks her old friend for a way to talk directly to the people affected by the outbreak. The very next day, Melissa announces that they will hold a kitchen cabinet meeting in the St. Peter's rectory. Apparently, Melissa believed that the rectory would offer appropriate privacy, and that the kitchen cabinet—like those of former presidents—could give advice discreetly and in confidence, with no more responsibility or authority than they would have as private citizens.

Now, Connie greets the women as they enter like she greeted guests in the receiving line at her wedding reception. Melissa introduces each and Connie remembers what she can from when she and Melissa identified whom they would invite and what they would be discussing. The agenda they have before them is like a television guide in which each stakeholder is a channel, and they will—if a channel isn't working—change channels as needed.

First to arrive is Suzy, the representative of the parent group. Bright, warm, personable, and dressed for success in a blue suit and white blouse with frills showing at the cuff, she holds her hands together over her navel in a prim gesture that pushes her shoulder purse back a bit too far. Despite her engaging look, and the way her shiny black curls fall neatly around her shoulders, Connie notices immediately that her eyes are too close together, her thumbs are too broad, and her left ear looks like it was mutilated by a graduate of the School of the Americas—three dysmorphic features visible at first glance.

What Connie can't see, and what Melissa hasn't told her, is that Suzy has had two children and four abortions, all of the latter for conditions that would have been fatal to the child had the pregnancy continued past the first trimester. What Connie can see, when she is done with her quick and hopefully discreet visual examination, is that Suzy has presented her beauty in such a way as to charm even those like Connie who can't look past the flesh.

Suzy also has something that most people see without recognizing it—a glow of love that reminds Connie very much of Brother Ben. And Connie can tell from Suzy's smile that she is not faking this glow. She has grappled with despair and found her way to an inner light that can never be extinguished. Suzy is the wild card, the unexpected resource that comes into every meeting. In this case, she is the navigator through tight emotional spots. Connie always looks for such facilitators, but never counts on finding one. Connie only hopes that Suzy's mind is as open as her heart.

Then it is Helen who arrives, the Sierra Club representative and activist in more groups than Connie can remember. Helen will be easy to identify because she looks like she is about to chain herself to a tree in a vain effort to show loggers that live trees have more value than cut ones. Helen wears hiking boots, pants frayed here and there by jagged rocks and thorny scrub, and a thin T-shirt that shows businesslike biceps and a lithe form suggesting a high level of cardiovascular fitness.

With a pretty, green-eyed, freckled face framed by wavy strawberry blond hair, Helen is the picture of health and boundless optimism. But Melissa, and now Connie, both know that Helen has had two miscarriages, and is addressing her grief by devoting herself to protecting all unborn souls. She does this by guarding the bounteous mother of all mothers, Gaia, the Earth herself, from the creeping death doled out by chainsaw blades, distant landmines, and the scouring of bulldozers. It is Helen who is Connie's greatest fear because she is both an example of self-sacrificial integrity and a reminder that the life within Connie's womb, the life she now loves more than her own, is fragile and could disappear at any moment.

Next to arrive is Jennie, the environment reporter from the Denver Dispatch whose presence is a complete surprise, with makeup applied so thickly that Connie has no real idea what she looks like. It's as if Jennie is wearing a disguise that will enable her to go incognito just by washing her face. Wearing a tight dress that would reveal her shapely figure to anyone who might belly up to a bar, what neither Melissa nor Connie knows is that Jennie had a wild time in the sixties, during which she picked up a sexually transmitted disease that traveled up her intrauterine device to her fallopian tubes and ovaries, leaving her infertile. She has never told anyone, except her ex-husband—who promptly left her—and prefers the lie that she never wanted to have children. This story makes her feel powerful, and able to ignore the scars left on the most private parts of her body.

Connie isn't quite sure *how* she knows, but sees with a shock of recognition that Jennie lacked a father. She can't tell, yet, exactly what form of lack it was, but she feels certain Jennie has provided herself with yang energy by drawing on a store that was always too small. She protects, or perhaps conceals, with an edge designed to put others off; and her makeup is another form of concealment rather than an attempt to allure. Connie is fairly sure that if they have to do something difficult or hurtful, Jennie will be the one to call on: She too is a reluctant warrior.

When the three early birds have all perched at the dining room table, and Mrs. Hernandez is bringing them coffee, Pat, the computer whiz and information technologist representing the Department of Health, arrives. According to Melissa, Weinstein sent Pat as a snub because she has next to no rank at the Department, but if that is the case, the joke is on him because he has sent the one person in his group who knows *exactly* what cold facts his department can and can't provide. An easy-going, dispassionate, and attractive woman with no need for attention, admiration, or concealment, Pat dresses simply, says little, and maintains a warm quiet that is like a pleasant forcefield of calm reason. Her features are regular and symmetrical, her hair an indefinite brown. Connie fixates immediately on Pat's most striking characteristic, her height, which she guesses is six feet.

Pat is also the department psychologist, the one who can hold anyone's hand when the hardware fails, or the software frustrates. She is also the one who gets warring departments to pay attention to the fact that to get what they want, they will have to agree on certain reasonable things. The arbiter of the playground, she is the child who calms others by staying calm herself. And what Melissa knows, but Connie doesn't, is that Pat comes from the kind of family that would take her to the emergency room for strange behavior because she is the only one of her relatives who is not seriously disturbed.

Kathryn, the Episcopal priest who represents a neighborhood near to Melissa's, arrives last looking harried and in need of a confession. Once she takes a seat at the table and begins to calm down, she turns into a sphinx. The politician of the group, she is the one who speaks out of calculation and, perhaps, cunning.

When Connie has met them all, and they have taken seats around the lace-laden table in the rectory dining room, she has the sinking feeling that this meeting is actually a very bad idea. She is especially worried about upsetting the member of the parents' group, even though Melissa is satisfied that Suzy is ready because her child is well past the crisis stage and thriving. Connie fears that even in this tiny crucible, Dr. Cowan will be proved right that what people want to hear, above all, is that everything is under control. She is reluctant to throw a rock at the big bad barrier of denial in case they decide to shoot the messenger—or burn her for a witch.

She pulls Melissa aside. "Why are they all women?"

"Are they? I didn't notice."

"Oka-a-a-ay."

"I just invited the stakeholders who I thought would be best able to tolerate ambiguity."

"What about Suzy? The mom. She has dysmorphic features."

"No more than the rest of us. Remember, everyone has two or three."

"Not in this context."

"What do you mean?"

"I mean it's reasonable to infer that her child has a genetic condition, which means that her inclusion in the outbreak investigation is an accident of geography, and a mistake."

"First of all, you don't know whether there might have been a contributing factor, like a toxin or infection. Second, just because you can't see susceptibility in the others doesn't mean it isn't there. And third, her kid faces the same issues as the others. It wouldn't be fair to exclude her."

Once they are all assembled around the table, Connie quails, wishing it was just Melissa so she didn't have to tell this group that she has no real good news for them. She tries to take heart from the fact that they are all women, and as such may be subliminally aware that fertility has been endangered by the great economic machine which is a limp substitute for the human heart and mind, and that more and more upwardly mobile couples have few skills and little time for parenting. Then Connie realizes, with a shock, that she herself believes she should be completely devoted to the happiness of her own family.

She also realizes that she should say why they are meeting at the rectory, which was offered by Father Sean as neutral ground. Helen looks as if she is about to be sick; Jennie is making frantic notes as she steals dark glances at the lurid, bloody, crucifix above the head of the table; while Pat—who it occurs to Connie, is probably a former Catholic—is sitting a pace away from the table with her arms crossed. Even Kathryn, the Episcopalian priest, looks a bit apprehensive.

But Melissa seems oblivious, and Suzy is the only one who seems to feel at home. Connie decides to open up to this group as much as she can, and so set the stage for radical trust. She gets up, gathers her determination and courage, closes the door, and proceeds to start by telling them some of her own secrets.

9

Home

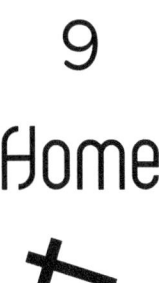

Connie draws strength from the mountains. She felt nothing for them as a child, barely noticing them in the background of the swing set or the baseball diamond, but now they feel like home.

As the road veers east between the foothills and heads toward the wrinkled, tree-whiskered face of Mount Princeton, Connie is awed by its titanic glory, and unexpectedly moved to tears. Back in college, she had been torn between the quiet cocoon in which she'd lived with her mother in Alamosa and the jostling world of ideals and chaotic details in Boulder that all demanded attention and allegiance. Now, turning on the road to Alamosa, she once again feels the inner warmth and simplicity she knew while cooking dinner as her mother did the ironing; or sat at the kitchen table doing homework while her mother knitted or mended, feet swinging under the chair, bathed in invisible love. At the same time, she feels a surge of anger at Pippie for forcing this visit to her mother, the one person in the world most likely to inadvertently shatter her resolve—the one whose inability to talk about her father could still trigger Connie's fears and doubts.

Torn between anxiety and love, she watches the Sangre de Christos Mountains reach ahead on either side like arms holding the flat expanse of the San Luis Valley. She can see Alamosa, now, and imagines Conejos County and New Mexico like a mirage beyond it. As the road descends into the Valley, which seems to embrace the deep blue evening sky, both anxiety and love resolve into concern as she realizes that she is ready—even eager—to care for her mother.

Connie's eyes drink in the view of the mountains on the left, which form a line of gigantic deep maroon cones of perfect beauty, and those on the right, which draw the valley's distant, purple edge. At Mosca, where the mountains disappear and leave only a broad, desert plain, Connie begins to cry again. Laced through her mother's love are painful cords of sorrow that could constrict at any time, and bind the two of them together in a way that excludes the joy and ease Connie has found with Pippie. Her mother is quick to feel hurt, and will probably feel devastated that Connie did not mention her visit to Colorado.

Connie tries to prepare for her mother's sorrow, and to extinguish the persistent and unreasonable hope that her mother may, just this once, tap into the wisdom of the peaceful and knowing heart hidden deep inside her. Then she may see Connie's troubles, and be able to provide the irreplaceable parental gift of dispassionate wisdom and advice. Things will be okay in any event: Connie will be able to do it even if her mother can't.

By the time Connie approaches Alamosa, the sky is dark except for a line of blue on the horizon. As the carpet of town lights spreads out on either side of the highway, twinkling and promising the refuge of home, she is glad to be arriving at night when she can feel that the only part of the town that matters is her mother's tiny apartment. Her feelings are mixed, but settled, when she imagines herself entering the living room, with its persistent smell of simmering peppers, and hearing the sound of the television punctuated by the hiss and whoosh of her mother's steam iron.

Then, as her mind's eye brings the collection of second-hand porcelain knick-knacks on the shelves above the television stand into view, Connie remembers how as a small child she longed to touch them, but her mother had refused to bring them down. When she was old enough to reach them herself, and therefore to be trusted to handle them with care, she discovered that each held a story that changed as her imagination grew. By the time she visited home as a medical student, she was slightly ashamed of her lingering affection for what she came to see as cheap and sentimental tchotchkes. Eventually they became symbols of her identity as the child of an unwanted refugee and the illegitimate child of a sinful priest. Because her mother was attached to them, Connie had coped by pretending that the figures no longer meant anything to her.

Parking in front of the grand old mansion that had once housed a Mormon family, and is now subdivided into apartments, Connie steps into the welcome chill of evening—which smells slightly of garbage. After stretching her legs under the lone streetlight, she pulls her bag out of the trunk and walks across the gravelly lawn toward the garage in the back, tripping on the stump of a tree that was cut down since her last visit. At the screen door of the garage apartment, Connie stops to listen for sounds of her mother, but hears only the television. Uncertain whether to knock, which is overly formal, or to walk in, which may frighten her mother, Connie finally knocks and then calls out.

Receiving no response, a frightened Connie opens the door, dragging her bag into the sooty, cramped kitchen. Going into the living room beyond, she is relieved to find her mother in the reclining chair below the black velvet picture of a kitten, staring at the old television. Mama's eyes are red behind her horn-rimmed bifocals, and her nose sniffles as her big-knuckled fingers work a wrinkled handkerchief. Mama is so much heavier than she was four months ago that Connie's first impression is of a short Sumo wrestler in a green and red flowered housecoat and red scuffs. Without looking at Connie, her mother says in her lightly accented English, "You shouldn't come. I'm just a burden to you."

Connie's relief vanishes. She feels again the heavy weight of responsibility for the welfare of her mother, and in turn of the world. That weight long ago seeped into her bones, like poisonous salts of heavy metals that are now and then released. "Ma, I have a lot of responsibility right now," she says, sitting down with her purse still in her hand. Her mind races to make things right. "Didn't you see me on TV?"

The television is the third member of their little family. Her mother glances at Connie and puts down her handkerchief. "Were you on TV?"

"I was on the news talking about those children with the birth defects. We're trying to find out why they were born that way. But we've run into problems."

"Those poor mothers! Are you helping them?"

"I hope so, Mama. I'm trying." *Easier to take on the sorrows of the world than try to stop your tears*, she thinks. "Is there anything to eat? I'm starved."

Mama climbs to her feet and shuffles toward the kitchen, scuffs dragging. "I have your favorite. Spaghetti!"

Connie can't remember ever liking spaghetti, but seeing her mother happy, responds cheerfully, "Perfect! Thanks."

When they sit together at the round Formica table beside the television, Mama drinking her evening mug of hot water and Connie eating her spaghetti, her mother observes, "You look so healthy! You were too thin."

"You know how Pippie likes to eat."

"I had a period yesterday! I haven't one for years. Isn't that strange?"

"It certainly is." *Maybe I should have one.* An impulse to change the topic makes it easier to say, with a somber expression, "Ma, I've got to ask you something."

As her mother fiddles with the string tie of her housecoat and stares at the table, Connie worries that Mama's eyes are getting red, but still chooses to speak.

"I want to see my father. You don't have to come, but I want to meet him and talk to him."

Ma's lips begin to tremble. "You can't see him."

"Ma, you always said that when I was ready, I could visit him. I would have asked ten years ago, but I didn't want to upset you."

"We waited too long, little bird," Mama weeps. "Father O'Reilly died. And now you can never meet your earthly father."

"What did he die of? How old was he?"

"God took him, little bird, when he was ready."

"Oh, Ma! Did you keep the obituary? Do you know the date?"

"Father Polaski told me. That's all I know. That's all I know. I forgave him and now I don't want to think of him again. You have your mama, and a Father in heaven."

Connie bites her lip, which bleeds slightly, and swallows the flood of her feelings in order to pay attention to her mother's. "Pippie thinks you should come live with us, Ma. You can't stay here by yourself anymore. You worked enough in your life."

"I can't leave my church," Mama asserts, gripping her mug as if clinging to the familiar. She had resolved her crisis of faith by deciding that Father O'Reilly, the rapist, and his parish, who ostracized her in a most un-Christian way, were an anomaly, a den of sin that proved the need for the larger church. She had turned to a parish in the rival town of Conejos, where she was welcomed and given sympathy and understanding. With the help of Father Polaski in Conejos, and the Mormons in Alamosa, who gave her work as a laundry woman, she and Connie had survived—and thanks to Great Society scholarships, even thrived.

"You can come back and visit them," Connie says.

"I would never leave," Mama insists. "Except, of course, for a grandchild."

Connie is not ready to reassure her mother on that score, not before the amnio. It will be months before she knows that the fetus may be viable. "I ought to get to bed now," she says with unfeigned exhaustion. "I have an early breakfast meeting. Do you want me to get some groceries and make that tuna casserole for you before I go?"

"You won't be here tomorrow?"

"I might be able to get back for lunch. Don't wait for me, though. It depends on how everything goes." Connie stands and gives her mother a long hug, bending awkwardly so as to keep her belly at a distance. Dragging her suitcase to the back room that holds the laundry machines, she sees the old washer with a mangle, and, behind lines of drying linens, two narrow single beds, Connie smiles to think of Pippie trying to sleep in one of them.

"Are you coming, Ma?"

"Okay." They take turns putting on their nighties and brushing their teeth in the little bathroom off the laundry room, and then go to bed. Instead of falling asleep, they lay in the dark and chat for an hour about linens, recipes, television shows, and Mama's friends in Conejos County.

At ten o'clock the next morning, Connie is still waiting in the downtown pediatric clinic to meet Dr. Alex Taub. She could have waited at her mother's home, only a few blocks away, but didn't want her mother to detect her morning sickness. She had been able to put the time to good use, however, first when Dr. Taub was delayed by a case of nursemaid's elbow, and then by a case of anaphylactic shock following an insect bite. When the staff gave Connie an empty back office from which to make calls to verify, or exclude, cases reported from Telluride and Durango, she was unusually lucky in confirming or excluding all but one case—and one case would not be enough to justify a trip. After meeting with Dr. Taub, she will be free to stay with her mother and to return to Denver in the morning.

Connie yawns and swivels back and forth in her wheeled desk chair as she drafts a report based on the notes made during her telephone calls. When she finishes, and is considering what to do next, a young doctor with a dark cowlick sweeps in with a broad smile, sits on the examining table, drapes his stethoscope behind his neck with a flourish, and leans back on one arm. He pulls in his chin, composes his features into a look of impenetrable confidence, and stares down at Connie expectantly.

Connie suppresses a smile. "Thank you for your time, Dr. Taub. I know you have patients waiting, so I'll get right to the point. I need more diagnostic information about the cases reported to the Health Department. It turns out that some of the cases reported as having midline facial defects had only cleft lip and palate. I'd be happy to review your records if you don't have time."

"I'm afraid I can't help. I don't make the final diagnosis. I refer all my cleft cases to Dr. Kazanjian. He's the expert."

Connie sees herself jumping up and scolding the young doctor. But even as her face turns red, and beads of sweat appear at the young man's hairline, she is flooded with an odd and unexpected tenderness for the hapless young doctor. Taking a deep breath, she begins slowly, looking at the ceiling as she tries to find the words.

"They don't teach you this in medical school, but surgeons, except for general surgeons, depend on primary care doctors like you to make the diagnosis. Surgeon's diagnoses are affected by what we call a "referral filter." In other words, they see cases that have already been labeled and sorted, so they don't really know what to do with a full spectrum of cases, and tend to over-diagnose. It's critical that you be the diagnostician *and* the filter, especially at a time like this when the general community is so upset and concerned that people are seeing cases everywhere. You are qualified to make the diagnosis simply by looking at the patient."

Connie reaches forward and pulls a photocopy of a textbook page from her briefcase, handing it to Dr. Taub. "The lines on this diagram show Tessier's classification of facial clefts. We are looking for midline defects only. It's quite simple."

Dr. Taub holds the paper between his thumb and finger, but doesn't look at it. "Dr. Kazanjian is an accomplished surgeon and professor. I'm sure I can depend on him."

Ordinarily, the implication that Connie doesn't know what she is doing would infuriate her, but even though this doctor is only a few years younger and a good deal taller, his youthful ignorance and insecurity strike her as poignant.

"You shouldn't expect him to do your part of the work and his part too. The surgery is a difficult and treacherous. It's enough!"

"He was my professor."

"You were the student then. You're the doctor now." As he studies the diagram, Connie is tempted to say, just between you and me, the fact that your Dr. K. can't be bothered to do his work may account for the whole crisis—but she can see that would be too harsh. This young man needs to gain confidence in himself, rather than lose confidence in Dr. Kazanjian. "Does that make sense?"

"Sure. It's just that the MS Center wants their cases to be confirmed by specialists, so I assumed you wanted the same thing. It would be easier if you guys had one form."

"One form?" Connie taps her pen distractedly on the desk at her elbow. "What—a multiple sclerosis outbreak?"

"Oh, Christ! This is too much. You government guys always come down here and tell us what to do, but you never know what's going on!"

"Did anyone from the Health Department contact you about the MS outbreak?"

"Yeah, I got a letter from, what's-his-name, Weinberg."

"You mean Weinstein?"

"Yeah. Weinstein. Ira Weinstein."

Connie exhales, puffing out her lips, and then gurgles out a long, slow cackle. "Will the wonders of bureaucracy never cease? I'm sure Weinstein never thought for one moment of anything other than labeling and sorting: CDC investigation here, University research there. Birth defects here, neurological diseases there. There is another, more fundamental step that we have to take before labeling and sorting."

"What are you mumbling about?"

"Look, what do we doctors do? Diagnosis, prognosis, and treatment, all based on pathology and ultimately anatomy, with a little physiology thrown in. But to practice prevention, we have to look at things differently."

"What do you mean?"

"We have to step back and ask ourselves what the coincidence of these two outbreaks might mean. For one thing, we have to ask if it's the same outbreak!"

"That's ridiculous! One's a malformation, and the other's an immune disorder."

"That's what most people would say. Weinstein had the same mindset, which is why he never connected the dots to put the two investigations together. They were so far apart in his mind he didn't even notice the administrative advantages of combining them. But that mindset is wrong. One cause can have many results."

"You sound like the environmentalists."

"Did they say the outbreaks might be connected?"

"Yeah, but they don't understand the medical realities. I mean, you can't just say, 'anything's possible.' You have to go with the science."

"Yes, but this is the science. We're facing the unknown with both these outbreaks, and we have to be open-minded and apply reason to our observations, not cling to faulty preconceptions and stereotyping. Think about it. We've known for millennia that one cause can have many results. Strep infections can cause acute glomerulonephritis and rheumatic heart disease. TB is the same way. Remember what they used to say about syphilis? He who knows syphilis knows medicine? It can cause virtually anything. And especially remember rubella. It causes measles in the mother and birth defects in the baby. What if a virus went through here that caused clefts in fetuses and MS in adults?"

"But it takes years for MS to develop."

"That's good reasoning, unless the pregnant mothers' infections are chronic."

Dr. Taub frowns and stares at the window above Connie's head, then looks at his watch. "All this philosophizing is great, but I have to see a patient. Let me know what I can do."

"You could use the Tessier system in your diagnostic notes."

"Sure, but that won't help with the old cases."

"Right. Might there be any photos or diagrams in those charts? If there aren't, I'll try talking with the mothers. I should be talking to them anyway."

Dr. Taub stands up, folds the diagram, and slips it into his pocket. "Thanks for this sheet. You're welcome to look at the charts. Do you have a card?"

"Yes. Feel free to call me or Dr. Gomez if you have any questions." Connie hands him a card from her purse.

"Not Dr. Weinstein?" he asks with a mischievous smile.

Connie makes the motion of zipping her lips. "I'll have Dr. Gomez clarify the reporting system in his press release, and I can't promise anything, but I'll see what I can do to instigate a combined reporting form."

As Dr. Taub leads Connie to the shelves of records behind the reception desk, she calculates the number of hours it should take to see the case mothers, who live all over the valley. She would have to stay another day, which means more time with Mama. Her heart warms—and then cools with the thought that this also means more chances for her mother to discover her pregnancy before Connie is ready to tell her about it.

Connie can't believe that the men and women who work the potato fields all week come to this hall and dance for hours straight. They are dynamos; tough and fit and vital. The statisticians who have declared them poverty-stricken because they live largely outside the cash economy know nothing of culture or spirit or place.

The food laid out on the side table has enough peppers in it to keep the sauce makers in Louisiana busy for weeks. When the *abuelas* fuss over her, she pretends to dislike it, but inside she feels like the belle of the ball, of the *quinceañera,* the coming of age party at which she would have danced with her father—had she had either the party or the father.

Her mother, who always seems to her to be mousy, has been spinning like a prima ballerina with several men young enough to be her sons, and several old enough to be her father.

To an outsider, it might look like a lively but poor affair, but Connie's practiced eye sees the richness. She sees the hairdo that took an hour, the embroidery that represents weeks of work, the makeup that was nearly too expensive to buy. She sees the care and love that the community has put into this.

She feasts her eyes on the beauty of this moment, and savors its details: Bored concertina player. Plump vocalist. Flying fiddle bows. Energy in the room. Heat like a warm fire. Enchilada torte. Chimayo rug underfoot. A few Mormons in one corner, tall Spanish-speaking Indians, a couple of Mexicans, and her Bolivian mother. Everything in the hot room spinning. It's amazing how quickly they dance without bumping into each other. Connie's mind starts to devise a mathematical equation to describe their movement.

Then she sees a woman snubbing her mother, and can see nothing else. Connie starts toward her mother, when she is stopped by an *abuela* who draws her to a cluster of smiling faces. "We saw you on television, *hija,* you have become a big celebrity!"

And then their faces radiate sorrow as concern pours out of their eyes.

"Tell us, what will happen to those poor *niños?* You must find out what is causing this terrible thing!"

Connie answers dutifully and completely, and then, as more

people join the group and the questions become repetitive, she exits to the yard where she pulls out a large mobile phone from her pocket and dials. Noticing a line of drunken men in the shadows who are cursing each other in Spanish, and who don't seem to see her, she speaks freely, but in a low voice.

"Pippie? It's me baby," she says, sighing heavily. "I just called to say hi and hear your voice!"

"Where are you?"

"At the Friday night dance at the Martinez farm," she says with a sad sniffle.

"What's the matter Pea?" he asks with alarm.

"It's great to see Ma, but it's hard to be here." She tells him her troubles, mixing the personal and the professional. Finally, she gets to the nub of her distress. "I don't know how to keep going. I'm losing my faith in life, Pippie. I don't know what I'm doing."

"Come home! Let Ramón finish the work."

"This should be my home too, but they want to pretend everything was fine—and it wasn't! How can I forgive the past when they don't even ask me to?"

"Your home is with me, Pea."

"Oh, that means so much to me! With your love and support—"

"Stop doing this work. Please, Pea. This new game is going to sell, and you'll be able to do whatever work you like. You can have kids, and your ma can come and live with us."

Pea uses her free hand to cover her mouth as she stifles a sob. "I wanted to forgive my father the priest and be forgiven for my anger, but I waited too long Pippie. He died!"

"It might be for the best. He might have disappointed you. Again."

"It must have been hard for him here. He must have heard

the most blood-curdling confessions—day after day, month after month, year after year. Maybe they dragged him down the way they dragged us down."

"You can't forgive a person if you don't hold them responsible."

"You're right, Pippie. You're right. But the people here loved him. He must have had some good in him."

"Of course he did. He fathered you. And he will be the grand-father of our baby, and we'll want to tell her—or him—the good things."

Connie watches the men misbehaving. One pulls a knife as he staggers. She is sad for him, and a little afraid. Reaching deep inside, she releases her anger, then decides to give them a good scolding, crossed with a potent blessing. But first she will say goodnight to the father of her child.

"I love you, Pippie. I'm so lucky to have you in my life."

10
Rounds

"I know next to nothing about clefts, and this is our library," the young doctor says as he sweeps his hand dismissively toward the wall of books behind his desk chair. "I depend on specialists like Kazanjian."

Ramón suppresses his dislike of the young doctor, who is new to Eagle County and seems to resent questions. Having known hundreds of doctors, Ramón instinctively classifies them as defensive, which he dislikes; collegial, which he appreciates; collegial but protective, which he respects; or suspicious, which annoys him. He especially dislikes questions about his legal authority, partly because he doesn't know the answer, and partly because he thinks that moral authority should prevail. Fortunately, most doctors welcome him and understand that his main concern is their patients' (and the public's) welfare.

"For our purposes, it will be necessary to have as specific a diagnosis as possible in order to find the cause of the outbreak. Different clefts may have distinct causes."

"What makes you think there's a one-to-one relationship between cause and effect, or one cause per anatomical diagnosis?"

"In general, we expect causality to be specific."

"Nonsense. Smoking participates in the etiopathogenesis of a variety of diseases. And cancer, for example, has a variety of etiopathogeneses."

Ramón is momentarily unnerved, and then laughs. "You're absolutely right. We make assumptions and then forget them. But let me appeal to your common sense. Midline defects are rare, and not associated with cleft lip or palate. A cluster of midline defects is arguably an epidemic, an indicator that something new is wrong. If we don't identify those cases accurately, we won't know whether there's an epidemic."

"Something's always wrong," the young doctor retorts testily. But then he sighs, and braces his elbows on the desk to lean in toward Ramón. "Just between you and me, your partner is rubbing some people the wrong way."

"Connie? Dr. Martin?"

"She apparently caused a priest to have a heart attack."

"Speaking of causality, it's atherosclerosis that causes heart attacks."

"Don't neglect the precipitating factors. Look, whatever she may have done or not done, it could be a problem for you."

"Thanks," Ramón replies lightly, but then adds a more tactful explanation. "She's having some personal problems just now. I'll have a word with her. Thanks for telling me."

Inside, though, Ramón feels sick at the idea that she may have done something to stress a priest. After cordially concluding his interview with Dr. Piggott, Ramón goes to his rental car to finish his notes. Then, digging out a tiny black-covered book that Dr. Cowan gave him to record any public relations issues, he notes on its blank pages the incidents with Weinstein and the priest.

By the end of the day, he has visited all the practices except the one in Leadville. He has, so far, met five pediatricians who gave him full copies of beautifully detailed medical records; six family practitioners who shared very sketchy ones; an iconoclast who resented outsiders and the government, but resented Dr.

Kazanjian even more, and so gave Ramón nothing; a gregarious doctor who wasted an hour of Ramón's time with idle gossip and then couldn't find the patient's record; and a lonely doctor who implied that she would give him a record if he stayed for dinner. In the end, with the help of the operative and post-operative reports, he was able to classify the defects in all but three of the children.

Ramón goes to visit those three children in their homes, where he takes the opportunity to ask the mothers open-ended questions, listening carefully to their terse or rambling answers in search of a clue as to possible causes of the outbreak. The first two visits are uneventful, so much so that he can barely recall them the following day—but the last gets under his skin. It blindsides his ethics, and is likely to haunt him for a long time.

It is only by luck that Ramón finds the child, who lives in an isolated wood cabin set a mile above the winding mountain road to Leadville. If Ramón had lacked a good eye, or familiarity with topographical maps, he would have missed the peaked roof above the rocky outcrop on the forested slope—and also the overgrown rocky road that led up to it.

Swerving up the one-lane drive, hoping he won't meet another car, Ramón nearly gives up at every hairpin turn, half convinced he will be forced to back all the way down to the highway. He continues grimly, though, jaw clenched, until the road flattens and ends abruptly in a sunny clearing surrounded by tall, healthy pines.

The cloud of dust raised by his wheels leaves a gritty taste in his mouth and adds a fine layer of powder to the gray dust on the roof of the small brown cabin at the far edge of the clearing. Ramón worries for a moment that an unfriendly dog may bound out of one of the non-descript outbuildings on his right, but when he gets out of the car he hears nothing but the fan of his car engine and the rustling of the wind in the trees. He admires the spectacular view of the mountain ridges that define the valley below, reminding himself that a hundred years ago the whole region was a haven for consumptives fleeing cities and slums, and that he is too homesick to enjoy it. He is marooned in an alien place far from his many relatives, including the cousins who moved with him to Atlanta to fill his private life with all the love and responsibility he can manage.

The thought of finishing his work so that he can go home propels Ramón across the clearing and down the rough-hewn rock stairs to the screen door of the cabin. When he raises his hand to knock, he sees a woman looking at him from the shadows inside. She is tall, with sculpted cheekbones and long black hair woven into a thick braid that curves around her breast and dangles beside her waist. For a moment, he thinks she is his first love, Lucia. As she approaches the door, her large brown eyes look intently into his, and he feels Lucia's long hair brush his naked hips. The memory is so strong that he can only stare, open-mouthed, until she steps backward and asks guardedly, her hand at her throat, "Who are you?"

"I'm sorry, I couldn't see. You surprised me. Uh, Dr. Assad wasn't able to find your son's medical record and so I, um, I should introduce myself. I'm Dr. Gomez, from the Centers for Disease Control." He opens the door and extends his hand. "I'm here to investigate the birth defects out here. Your son is one of the children we can't classify with our records, so I wanted to see if I could examine him myself, if that's okay."

"He's not my son," she replies, touching his hand with her fingertips. While Ramón's mind is still caught in a meshwork of feelings, including a fear that she finds him intimidating, she adds, "His parents are gone."

"I see. Perhaps I should come back?"

"You'd better see him now, before our ride comes."

"I don't understand."

"I'm his aunt, eh. After Alex was born, his dad started drinking, and then he left. After I came up to stay with my sister, she left too. She went after him, I think, so I'm going to take Alex back to Shiprock with me."

"I'm sorry for your troubles," he says, feeling an entirely unprofessional and immoral urge to hold her.

She turns away abruptly, crossing the dark interior which is furnished like a sitting room, and standing beside a woven laundry basket balanced on a fraying, early American style couch. It takes Ramón a moment to understand that the baby is in the basket, and he kneels in front of the couch to peer inside. When his eyes adjust, he sees that the baby is alert, but quiet, and that his nose is flattened and marked down the middle by a long scar. He doesn't speak until he has examined the baby thoroughly.

"The defect is midline. Alex is definitely a part of our case group." He stands up, intending to look the woman in the eye, but his eyes fix on the braid that meets the delicate curve of her right clavicle.

"Dr. Kazanjian decided to close the cleft when he saw the family fall apart. He won't do the definitive procedure for several months."

"You speak like an expert," Ramón said.

"I'm a nurse," she states calmly. "I know what this looks like to you."

Ramón sees himself letting go and taking her right then, on the floor. He can feel the abundance of life pressing him to unite with her body—and in so doing triumph over death and loss, failure and despair. He can feel her heat, her breath, her heartbeat, her belly. The image is so intense that he doesn't register what else she has said until after he has followed her distractedly to the door.

"You know what? I can tell what you think, eh, by the look on your face."

He backs out onto the front stoop. *"Vaya con Dios."*

Ramón runs to the car and drives too fast down the narrow road, raising a cloud of dust that gives form to his confusion. He tells himself that he is relieved that the woman didn't understand his desire, which was embarrassing and unprofessional, and that his odd behavior led her to infer prejudice instead. He hadn't even asked her name. Even so, he cannot make sense of the visit. His feelings remain intense but unformed, filling an uncomfortable gap in his sense of himself. It isn't until Ramón reaches the outskirts of Leadville that he realizes he is sad and lonely, frustrated and helpless—a state he has nearly forgotten, but which has crept back over him in the enforced isolation of fieldwork.

He wants a wife and a family, but not yet. He sighs and decides to sleep with Chris, the blond EIS officer, as soon as he returns to Atlanta. They understand each other implicitly. By the time Ramón pulls up at the curb outside the Schultz house, his confidence has returned.

Patty Schultz greets him warmly, but Hector, who is squirming wildly in her arms and pounding her cheek with his head, wails his disapproval. Theirs would be a difficult interview for the average field officer, but Ramón, a born pediatrician nostalgic for the warm chaos of family life, thrives on it. When Patty telephones the other mothers, several come over with their babies, and he finds himself comforted in his loneliness, while at the same time receiving all the information he needs.

Patty and the others describe all of the children in detail, and show him pre-operative photographs of most of them. They have done detective work of their own, which they are happy to share with him. They have pictures, calendars, journals, albums with news clippings and hospital souvenirs, and heartening pictures that show some of the children after they are well healed.

Ramón has forgotten the ultimate purpose of his visit, until Patty speaks in a sad voice to Elaine, the mother of a recovered toddler who is sitting in a portable playpen.

"Lainie, Claudia's closing the aerobics studio for good."

"It's about time," Elaine replies. "Who needs aerobics around here? Don't give me that look, Patty. Even you said you'd rather be skiing! You only went there to support Claudia. We all did. Our deliveries ended her business."

"You did aerobics during your pregnancy?" Ramón asks as casually as possible, his heart racing. For the first time, he sees a pattern. The aerobics studio. The skis in the hallway. The altitude. Low oxygen plus an oxygen-demanding pregnancy plus oxygen-demanding exercise could equal too little oxygen for the baby. The questioning of old-fashioned ideas about pregnancy has led to many, many changes. Women are exercising during pregnancy, even at high altitude. This could explain everything.

"Yes! We did everything we could to make sure we had healthy babies!"

Ramón nods, thinking, *If only we knew how that was done.* He gets through the rest of the visit on sheer professionalism, and in the end feels confident that he is not imposing his personal doubts and feelings on Patty and the other mothers, even though he sees everything differently now. It is as if he has entered another dimension where light and shadow are in higher contrast, where the sunlight makes the lace curtains blindingly bright and the shadows of the heavy antiques darker and deeper.

At the first opportunity, he draws the meeting to a close. Departing, he walks with deliberate slowness down the front walk, then turns back to wave at the women standing on the front porch of Patty's home, their children around them. Ramón sees the lines on their faces and the weight of sorrow on their shoulders more clearly than before. He drives away from the house, but just before leaving town, pulls into a gas station where he slowly fills his tires with air so as to have time to think.

Kneeling on the ground there, he looks around again and again in case a car might leave the usual path of traffic and accidentally—or intentionally—hit him. He feels the presence of hazard. The invisible and the unknown, which he never blocks out or avoids, now seem to hold a sharper sense of menace. Even in the comfort and warmth of the Schultz living room, in the heart of those new families, he had been chilled by the vision of an unexpected and dark possibility: In trying to provide for their children in the very best way they could imagine, those mothers may have actually damaged them. He wonders if they, and he, have taken too much of the responsibility for their own health and wellbeing away from God and onto their own shoulders. Were they all, in this modern age of control and investigation, engaged in a great act of hubris?

On the other hand, he knows that the world is not designed around the limited understanding of any individual or group, least of all himself. His own horizons had obviously been too narrow. He had been afraid to open his eyes to all of the possibilities, had not accepted that light is defined by shadow, and that any action taken in the world, however well-intended, must have unanticipated consequences. It must yield a variety of aftereffects, each of which may be evident or hidden to an observer; and if evident, seen as good or evil. There is a hidden blessing in that broader view—evil and neutral actions yield good ends along with bad ones.

That notion is all very well and good, but what is he going to tell the mothers? Can he tell them that they may have hurt their children? Doing so after the fact would only engender pointless and harrowing self-recrimination. On the other hand, he has a responsibility to prevent harm to the unborn, to warn young women who might be pregnant of the possible hazards of exercise at altitude. The responsibility weighs on his chest; he puts down the air hose and stands with his hands on the hood of the car, breathing deeply and deliberately, trying to sort out his thoughts.

Moral issues are much simpler in the clinic, where he has only one goal: to do his best to help each and every patient navigate the dangerous, frightening, and often unpredictable path of illness. Now he has to consider patients who don't yet exist.

Doctors in clinics see only a piece of the puzzle, as do researchers looking for clues by which to increase medical knowledge; politicians who are responsible for making policy; and members of the public whose sense of safety may be bolstered, or crushed. He understands why his superiors are so concerned about public opinion: It affects the public welfare. When the time comes to draw conclusions, he will have to weigh every word he writes. He might have to be courageous and compassionate, bold and subtle. He will have to draw on the experience of others. And he will have to depend on Connie.

Before he makes any statements, he must reduce his uncertainty as far as possible. He has to be clear and precise. Hypoxia has been associated with birth defects, but not this pattern of defects. He mustn't jump to conclusions.

Ramón finishes filling the tires, which had plenty of air before he started, and then gets back in the car to drive more cautiously than usual back to Denver. He can't wait to see Connie.

When he finds her at her health department desk, and tells her what he suspects in the most uninflected and factual manner that he can muster, he can see that she, too, is excited, and is attempting to keep a lid on it. "Good work! I expected as much."

"How do we approach the possible discovery of a cause in the course of an investigation?"

"This is when the numbers become especially critical. We first have to refine our case counts and compare our rate with the Atlanta one, to make sure that we have the generally accepted evidence for an outbreak. We should exclude any cases that we can't verify, and scan for like clues in our copies of the case records."

"Perhaps." Ramón stretches out in the small chair next to Connie's desk, folding his hands behind his neck and leaning his head against the blue-carpeted wall. Gazing at the ceiling, he puts the huge knot of hair that is stuck behind Connie's left ear out of his mind—it reminds him of his sister's back when they were children and he'd stuck chewing gum in it. "We can limit the exclusions to those we know to have ordinary cleft. Some of the rest were diagnosed by conscientious dysmorphologists who would never misreport a facial cleft, some have pre-operative photos, some were confirmed with our medical record reviews."

"Is that information coded in your database?"

"Unfortunately, no. I didn't expect the Kazanjian problem."

"Let's tidy up the database."

Within a few minutes, they draw up a form and start to re-review their copies of the records. Connie pulls several hanging files from the box and opens one on her blotter. When they are halfway through, and have downed several cups of syrupy coffee from the urn in the small kitchen near the elevators, Connie sighs deeply. "Let's hope we don't lose too many cases. Our investigation will be over before it starts."

"Over?" Ramón asks absently.

"If we don't have enough cases, our findings won't be statistically significant, and we'll have to conclude that there was no outbreak."

"Dr. Cowan said that just *one* case could be considered an epidemic."

"He was probably talking about pneumonic plague. Something fatal that spreads."

"This is obviously an epidemic."

"Rare events often appear to cluster, but that can happen just by chance—or so we all assume. We can't raise the alarm unless we can show that chance is an unlikely explanation."

"Birth defects don't occur by chance. They have causes."

"Yes, but their causes are unknown, and those may cluster by chance. We have to have proof. Proof is what it takes to convince, and what will convince our colleagues that there's an epidemic is a statistically significant increase in rates. Even Father Sean expects this."

"Who?"

"He's … he's my confessor. And he's become like a surrogate father."

"Is he the one who had the heart attack?"

Connie puts her hand over her mouth. She can see Ramón's distress. She thinks of Missy's advice, and speaks only after a long pause. "There's a lot that I haven't told you. The first confession went badly, but we are becoming very close."

"Close?"

"I visit him at the rectory. He shares insights, gives me advice."

Ramón shakes off this unexpected revelation, and says a Hail

Mary in his mind. "Getting back to truth, what about common sense?"

"When you make a diagnosis, do you confirm it with common sense or lab tests?"

"This is different! We're here to protect the unborn. It's our job to find the truth. We can't let ourselves be diverted by faulty methodology. The burden of proof should be on disproving risk."

"In our culture money comes before life. Besides, we can only do what we can, which is less than we'd like it to be. Think it through. If the rates are so high that they can't be denied or explained away, we'll be forced to declare an epidemic; then we'll have to admit that we don't know the cause and can't control it, and all hell will break loose. Most people fear and loathe the unknown. They'll panic and blame us and the unborn will be as unprotected as ever, or worse, protected from the good along with the bad. And we'll have lost the public trust so that even if we do find something, our word will mean nothing."

While Connie continues to fill in her form, Ramón folds his hands behind his neck and stares at the ceiling again. He is so upset that it is several minutes before he can think, and several more before he can recall the presence of God in order to speak calmly. "People don't know what causes cancer, and they accept that. It's a matter of how it's explained to them."

"It's possible that an anecdote would be enough to justify a caution—at least off the record. Perhaps we can craft just the right magical sound bite." Connie pushes a blank sheet of paper next to the record on her blotter. "This nursing note describes the face in detail. I'll write it in the comment field and we can code it later."

Ramón sighs and goes back to his work. More than two hours pass before he realizes that his concentration is failing and that his neck has become stiff. He stands and stretches. Seeing Connie crouched over the desk, and the top of the maze of cubicles extending in all directions like the stalls of a barn, he feels a keen urge to see the sky. "I think I'll go across the street for a sandwich. You want anything?"

"No thanks. When we finish here, I'll take an early dinner."

After he's gone, Connie takes advantage of her relative privacy to call home.

"Hi, Pippie!"

"Pea? Your mom called. Her mind must be going—she wanted to know where you were. She's getting more like my mom every day. She shouldn't be there all by herself."

"Oh, Pippie, don't worry. I'm just so busy I can't spend as much time with her as she wants. There are clusters all over, and we may have to investigate more of them, and …"

"You're seeing someone, aren't you?"

"What?"

"You're keeping secrets from your mom, and you're probably keeping secrets from me. I knew all this travel would lead to trouble!"

"Oh, Pippie, I'm just overextended. Barely coping. These kids—I have dreams, Pippie. Nightmares."

"Is that what you were doing last night when I called?"

"I was out at Melissa's."

"Was that Ramón guy there with you?"

"Pippie, don't be ridiculous! I don't know where he was. I just want to be home with you." Connie chokes back a sob. "I just need a vacation."

"You need to quit that job. What's the point of doing something hard that people don't appreciate?"

"Oh, Pippie, that's why it's called public service. It isn't for fun."

"Come home now, Pea. I'll call your mom and tell her you're not feeling well."

"No, Pippie! She'd just worry. I'll call her. It'll be fine."

"I'm coming out there, Pea."

"Oh, Pippie. You barely go out. And think what it would cost for you to get two seats each way! We just need to hold on until I finish here. That's all."

"I don't like this, Pea. This doesn't feel right."

"Don't worry. We can talk more when I get home. Bye now. Kiss, kiss."

"Where'd you get that from? You never say that!"

"I don't know Pippie. Maybe I heard it somewhere. This visit is going on too long. I gotta wrap it up. I gotta go. Bye!"

11
Plans

✝

At four o'clock on Monday, one hour before Ramón is to send out his press release, he and Connie sit in her cubicle at the Department of Health, staring at each other across the desk. The wall to Connie's right is covered with sheets of yellow legal paper held up by push pins, each one showing a black ink diagram of arrows and boxes containing words like cleft, altitude, hypoxia, and exercise. On the wall behind her, more sheets of yellow paper show similar diagrams, along with words like virus, immune dysfunction, and effect modification.

"It's sheer speculation," Connie sighs, "all of it."

Ramón is too exhausted to be frustrated. "I should have sent out the press release hours ago. Days ago."

"Instinct tells me that your speculation is correct, but we'll never be able to prove it," Connie says, turning to stare at the curling yellow rectangles suspended behind her. "But even if we can't prove it, we can't in good conscience ignore it, either. Maybe we can tell the press that we have no evidence, and ask the kitchen cabinet to spread the word that high altitude and viruses, at least the ones circulating now, may be more dangerous than we knew."

"You want me to say that in the press release?"

"No! We can't say anything about our findings yet! We have to go back to Atlanta and present all our findings to Dr. Cowan. My guess is that he'll advise us to wait and see if any more cases come in, which would be good advice."

"So, I tell the press to wait and see?"

"No, you tell them we reviewed the reported cases and confirmed that there is a problem, but also discovered that doctors over-reported clefts to the Health Department. You clarify the case definition and point out that our case ascertainment differs from that of the MS Center. Then you drive me to the airport."

Ramón leans back in the chair and stretches out to full length with his hands folded behind his head. Feet nearly reaching the back wall of the cubicle, his elbows block the open doorway to his right, and a smile covers the width of his face.

"You look happy," Connie teases. "New luck with the ski town babes, I guess. You won't have to go back to that blonde bim—EIS officer, will you?"

"Connie—"

"Forget I said that. Whatever makes you happy, Raymond."

Ramón stands and stretches. "You should rattle my cage only *after* I write your press release."

"I shouldn't rattle it at all. I should rattle Weinstein's about his reporting system until he's annoyed enough to do a good job just to get rid of me."

"Is this what you're like when you're in a good mood?"

"Sorry to be a pain. I'm running out of gas. I'll have to turn into a desk jockey like Cowan, or quit and go into private practice."

"Just promise me you won't quit before we wrap this up."

"I promise. I feel heat coming, and it wouldn't be fair to leave you in it. Kazanjian's behavior is a problem—Weinstein had probably heard rumors, and was happy to get us in to stop him. Finding a cause would be research, and we're not allowed to do that."

"We're not allowed to discover anything?"

"Nothing new."

Ramón looks crushed.

Connie adds quickly, "At least we can protect patients and their problems from overtreatment. My guess is that as our X-rays get more detailed, that'll be a bigger and bigger problem for all kinds of conditions."

"That's not prevention. That's policing."

"That's why we wear uniforms."

Ramón replies pensively, "I don't see what we can do. K's got a really big ego, and he's got a lot to lose."

"Last time he got called on the carpet, he threatened to sue," Connie whispers.

"Last time?"

"He was reprimanded when too many patients showed up without admit notes. You see the pattern. He thinks his time is infinitely precious, and he can't stand spending any of it on work the little people can do."

"You wouldn't operate on a kid you'd never seen!" Ramón exclaims too loudly.

"No. But the point is, how do we get through to this guy and change his behavior?"

"He can't sue us for objecting to this!"

"Lawsuits are about money and power, and he has plenty of both. He's a surgeon! He gets sued for money all the time. He may feel that it's unfair, and he would be right."

"He must have a senior colleague," Ramón persisted.

"His mentor died a few years back," Connie explained, "and there are only two or three people in his field whose opinion he would take seriously."

"Wouldn't he listen to his patients and to other docs?"

"I doubt it. But this can't be the first time this type of thing has happened. There must be someone at CDC who's figured out how to handle it. I'm going to lob this back into Cowan's court."

"What do you mean?"

"This is a hot potato. We need the medical community behind us, and that's politics. And that's his forté."

"He knows his medicine, too."

Connie sighs. "He does indeed. I complain about him at times, and the way he uses me sometimes chills my bones, but he's good. I can't think of anyone else I'd rather work for."

12
Truth

C onnie looks dubiously at the menorah and the Christmas tree before saying to Melissa, "I thought Dan hated Christmas." "A lot of our friends celebrate the solstice, but I figure we should have a Jewish Yule."

"Is that ... a joke?"

"No! We Swedes kept *Jul* through a thousand years of Christian interference, and I'm not about to give it up now! I just want to back out the Roman influence and celebrate Jesus as a rabbi of his time."

Connie giggles. "You can't just pick and choose like that!"

"I believe what I believe. What else can I do?"

Standing, then heading for the door like a messenger who is being timed, Connie speaks with a sudden urgency. "I'm hot. I have to go out."

"Wait! It's freezing out. The warm winds won't melt the snow until tomorrow, or the day after."

"I have to cool off. Let's walk around the block."

"Sure, just—give me a minute."

Connie rolls her eyes and waddles outside to stand on the porch.

Melissa pokes her head out through the door, gear dangling from her free hand as if she were provisioning them from an outdoor supply store. "Do you want some pickles, or olives, or crackers?"

"I'd love some olives. How did you know?"

"Just a wild guess."

"Just a minute, though, I have to pee."

As Melissa opens the door for her, she says with a laugh, "This could go on all night."

When Connie returns, Melissa is bundled up and standing ready to help her into Dan's larger sized gear. After rolling up the sleeves and pantlegs, they amble up the front walk, then step carefully over patches of bare pavement and crunchy ice on the street. Dirty shrunken drifts, with patches of last season's brown grass, fill the side yard.

"I wish I hadn't told Pippie I was pregnant."

"I think he might have had an eentsy little bit of suspicion by now. At the rate you're going, you might even weigh more than him soon."

"I never thought he'd appoint himself manager of the pregnancy. He's bought all kinds of how-to books and videos. And he talks about them. All the time."

"At least he's looking forward to fatherhood."

"Yes. But where's the book that tells you how to love? I feel this love that melts me like wax, but burns me at the same time. And I don't—" Connie stops. Her eyes feel as big and wet as watermelons. "I don't know what it's like to have a father. Is he crazy, or is he normal?"

"He's normal. But why don't you ask Father Sean?"

"What would he know?"

"He's like your father now, isn't he?"

"He's a priest!"

"He's a man. I'm guessing he isn't called Father for nothing."

"They don't know anything about women's business—as Aussie aboriginals call it."

"My guess is that men the world over are just as clueless. But it won't be a problem if you realize that you know more than Pippie—or any other man, for that matter."

"That's easy for you to say. You have a father."

"I do. I have a great father. And maybe you could have one too."

"You can't just pick one."

"Why not? According to Claude Levi-Strauss, some cultures have kinship structures in which every man of the parent's generation is a father."

"He needs me, you know. Father Sean needs someone to keep him sharp. You could make the case that I'm his mother."

"Or his teenaged daughter."

"What can he possibly know about parenting?"

"Ask and find out."

The two friends circle the block of houses, each other, and the family and professional conundrums that dog the problem-solving pathways of their entangled minds.

At the third corner, Connie slips, holding her belly protectively as Melissa grabs her elbow, which could have caused a fall except that Connie leans into her friend. Together they find balance and safety.

"Know what? Pippie's down to 250 pounds!"

"That's fabulous! He's more than halfway to normal weight!"

"I hope he keeps going that way. The baby will be here soon!" Connie's brow furrows at the thought.

"Don't rush him. You know it isn't safe, or wise, to lose too much too fast."

"The weird thing is, I don't like it. I liked him the way he was. He was my rock."

"Think of it this way: he'll be able to corral the kid."

Connie unzips the jacket and pulls off the cap; walking is making her hot. Soon she will have to go in and sit still to cool off. She is cautious, now, about exerting herself here in Colorado—especially given that she is spending most of her time in Atlanta at low altitude. There, her superiors watch the political situation while she and Ramón draft the elusive narrative that they hope will neither avoid, nor overstate, their uncertainty. It is becoming all too obvious to them that their message must be clear, and that they will therefore be obliged to oversimplify the situation to the point of obfuscation.

Connie sighs as she continues. "It's not that simple. He was an ocean of calm. I liked closing my eyes and getting lost in him. He's different now. He's ... rambunctious."

Melissa laughs. "Oh, Pea. Change is always hard, but give it a chance. Give it a few years. Can you get your arms around him?"

Connie smiles. "Not yet."

"From now on, you'll have new challenges every year. I worry about having kids who reach puberty. That's when my father went missing. He just looked at my two little peas-on-a-board breasts and pushed me out of his life for good. He related to me sexually after that, and he dealt with it by not dealing with me at all."

"I didn't know your father had let you down! I usually see that in people right away. I almost always see that absence from my own experience of never having had a father."

"Never? I thought you said he left your mom when you were little."

"Easy to believe, isn't it? Takes it out of the conversation; that's why I say it. The truth is, he was never with my mom. I never knew him. And now he's dead, so I never will."

"Oh my God. I'm so sorry to hear that! And I'm impressed that you've told me."

Connie feels Melissa's questioning eyes boring into her. "I wouldn't have said anything if you hadn't surprised me just now."

"Family stories are like those in the original Torah: They all need to be redeemed. They need to be revitalized, and passed on as healing stories. And you've already begun to do that."

"How can I possibly tell my story as a healing one?"

"When you figure that out, you'll be a great mom. Or grandma. Take whatever time you need. Think of it as your life purpose. That's how I think of Dan's task. His father was awful, physically abusive. I don't know any details because Dan can't talk about it. It poisons our intimacy. Be sure to tell Pippie everything. You can tell me whenever, but he needs to know soon."

Connie replies with new confidence and diplomacy. "Medicine is redemptive. You can't help someone across the thresholds of life or death without seeing how much we have yet to learn."

"Some deny all of that, but you and I won't," Melissa declares optimistically.

"Dan will, and he had a father."

Melissa sighs. "Different people react very differently to the same trauma. Think of the vets who came back from Pacific war prisons deaf and broken, and made good in spite of it all; and the ones who saw very little action, yet went mad. I'm guessing Dan will never heal—but I hope you will."

"Ramón's always talking about St. Paul's call to unceasing prayer. And always trying to do it."

"To live on his knees?" Melissa jokes.

"No! To be aware of the presence of God in every moment,

in every thought and every action. I need something else—a way of thinking that patterns the way I think and feel as a doctor and a mother. Something besides my mother's fears and an arbitrary list of dos and don'ts. I want to show my baby how to be; how to become; how to do."

"After the delivery," Melissa says facetiously.

"Yes, and no. I'm sure I'll change when I see the new life emerge. I may lose sight of the big picture that Father Sean and Ramón can see."

"You've certainly changed. You're more relaxed, you let your warmth and lightness show."

"I think we change from the inside, with the purpose and meaning of life, which for me is the responsibility of truth-telling for the sake of all children. I have to craft a message that lets people feel as if they can count on us for something other than politics, but we almost never get to the bottom of things, or protect the public from new epidemics. All we do is surveillance, and cloak it in PR."

"Pea, you and Ramón have been working on an investigation that goes far beyond PR. You're talking as if you knew what was wrong and were ignoring or hiding it. But you're up against the limits of human knowledge."

"My point exactly. We don't know much about birth defects. People either say, okay, well, there's really no problem because every child should be valued, or every child that isn't the way we want should be aborted."

"Really?"

"Yes. There's no constituency for preventing birth defects," Connie replies.

"I hope more of us will want us to try and see how we can prevent them."

"A hundred years ago, docs in obstetrics and gynecology asked themselves how to reduce infant and maternal mortality, and they did such a good job of it that we take it for granted now that childbirth will go well."

"Our old problems seem to be rare now, but we have new ones—like autism."

"And a high rate of infertility," Connie says. "We have no idea what Love Canal and other waste sites are doing to us—and our methods will never tell us."

"What do you mean?"

"Well, where we find a problem, we draw a big target around it. If that dilutes the problem, we then apply statistical methods of very low power and blame chance, as if it explained biomedical phenomena."

"It's hard to face events calmly."

"If you were a man, you could declare war on it."

"The war on heart disease, cancer, and stroke worked well. It makes sense to fight back, as if our health care system is like a big immune system," Melissa muses.

"That works only if we use strength rather than force. Force is just another weakness. Love and support feed the immune system; anger and fear undermine it."

"You *are* healing!" Melissa laughs.

"Maybe Cowan's right. Maybe everyone wants so much to believe everything's under control that there's no point in fighting it. Besides, NIH is supposed to do research, not us."

"It's risky to study real problems. You can fail. You can lose your funding and your job, and still accomplish nothing."

"It's interesting to watch Ramón wrestle with all of this. He likes things black and white."

"He's just starting out, isn't he? Must be overwhelming."

"And he's very, very Catholic. He wants to know God's truth, but he disapproves of ambiguity. In our line of work, that's like being a fish that disapproves of the ocean."

"I think it's all part of the bigger problems of complex systems. Things that are complex go wrong."

"Like the development of an embryo. I could have a child that needs my full attention all the time, and never have the chance to care for others."

"You mean a child with a birth defect?"

"Or a crier, or a preemie, or one that never sleeps. Or the baby may make very light demands. But I won't know until I see what the baby needs, how I feel, what I want to do, and what kind of help I can get."

"That's why you need faith."

"You're changing too." Connie smiles.

"I hope so. Stasis is death, and death should find no welcome here."

"Hear, hear. Now, let's go in and cool off." Connie begins removing her outer gear as she walks arm in arm with Melissa, wishing she lived closer to her old friend, to Father Sean, and to her hometown.

13

Atlanta

t's that surgeon," Dr. Cowan proclaims, his expression impassive. "He's created an outbreak of over-diagnosis and over-treatment. He drew attention to the problem, and now people are seeing it everywhere. You said that, and that's all you need in the final report."

"I don't think that accounts for the first cluster," Connie replies firmly.

Dr. Swanson, a skinny man of uncertain age with massive, white-blond eyebrows who is known for drawing a line in the sand and defending it as if it were a citadel, speaks dismissively. "You can't prove that there's an epidemic."

"You can't prove there isn't."

"It doesn't work that way."

"Maybe it should."

"But Connie, there's no evidence that this isn't a chance occurrence. This could all be bad luck. Bad luck happens, by definition."

"So does damage, by definition!" Connie declares.

"It's our job to evaluate the situation based on current knowledge and to recommend an intervention. It isn't our job to add to the fund of knowledge. We don't do research."

"We're lucky to have found a cause that we can eliminate," Cowan interjects.

Connie barely listens as Dr. Cowan repeats this rationalization for their many failures before she responds. "We *can* make the problems go away. We *can* set the criteria for proof so that nothing is ever proven."

Dr. Cowan frowns.

"We can't disregard the unknown, not when so little is known. Blissful ignorance is worse than panic. It sets us up for a catastrophic loss of confidence due to a pretense of innocence. That could lead to an epidemic of violence. The truth is that no one wants responsibility for reality—not you, not me, not the public. But it is officially our responsibility. When will we step up?"

"We are stepping up," Cowan disagrees. "We're taking responsibility for medical errors and preventing an epidemic of overtreatment."

"That, we can do on our budget," Swanson says. "It's practical."

Connie looks up at the panels in the old dropdown ceiling and wonders if they're made of asbestos. The truth is that the old portable building is decades past its expected life, the staff is underpaid, and even if their budget were ample, money could not buy the truth that awaits discovery.

She expected Dr. Cowan's calm disapproval. What she didn't expect was to be smiling, or to be feeling happy. She has, without even having researched or analyzed her situation, decided to quit and pursue her self-determined duty to speak for those who cannot speak for themselves.

"One case can be an epidemic," Connie continues. "The number of confirmed cases in affected counties is remarkable. This malformation is vanishingly rare, yet we have a large number of cases. The statistics are irrelevant. Of course, it would be cost-efficient and politically expedient to make it go away by diluting the rates through studying the whole state—an arbitrarily drawn area with no basis in biology. It's the only thing we can do, and should do. As long as we're not fooling ourselves."

Drs. Cowan and Swanson look at her and then exchange sharp glances. "Are the parents organized?"

"Yes," she replies. "The stakeholders are evenly divided between blaming the water and blaming God."

Cowan asks shrewdly, "And your one and a half?"

Connie is caught off guard and does not answer. She expected him to mention her condition right away or not at all.

"I found it difficult to do this work when my wife was pregnant; we're too aware of the risks. Have you decided what to do?" Cowan probes delicately.

"I'm going to have the baby, and return to the San Luis Valley to practice pediatrics part-time. I'd like this to be my last investigation."

Cowan raises his eyebrows, glances at Swanson, then says with feeling to Connie, "Well Connie, I'll be sorry to lose you. You keep us honest—with ourselves. But I respect your decision to quit. Family first. That's why we're here, to do what we can for families."

Connie smiles, then after a pause replies with a catch in her throat, "Thank you for saying that." She looks down at her notes and, finding her place, begins again. "And now, we have to do something about Dr. Kazanjian." She rubs her notes as if to clear away an invisible smudge. "We could put on a conference and invite him to talk about Tessier's classification of facial clefts, or we could ask him to be our consultant."

"I don't trust him," Swanson says.

"Neither do I," says Cowan. "Let's go with the conference. When you do your next press release, you can announce that you'll be inviting him to speak to all the key players."

"Shall we track down the missing cases?" Connie asks.

"If you have all the information you need on a town, skip it."

"I just want you to know that Ramón is the best I've seen."

"I'll make a note of your comment," Cowan promises.

"Okay, then. See you Friday." Connie's reply is quiet. She remains seated as the others take their leave, and she takes time to give thought to all that has transpired.

They have done everything right, to the best of their knowledge and ability, but there is a missing piece, something—or many things—they have yet to figure out. *There will always be things we don't know,* she thinks, *and there will be more and more as the radical, needless experiments of the modern era careen forward.* She entered the service with sanguine optimism, and leaves now with a superficial sense of peace, a deep foreboding, and prayers for whoever steps up to take her place. Their organization is the best in the world, yet it is doing far too little to discover what they must if they are to safeguard human life.

14
Vision

As usual, Ramón is out of bed and at his desk well before sunrise. He likes to do his prayer practice at three in the morning, when the world is quiet and his dreams have already brought him closer to God. At that time, he often slips quickly and deeply into the scriptural reading of the day, and feels that he may be coming nearer to putting on the mind of Christ.

Yesterday, Connie told him her story, and surprised him with her propriety—as well as her growing link with a priestly father figure. Ramón is able, for the first time in many months, to include her in his evening prayer with no sense of resistance, and to express his gratitude with new conviction. *We all do the best we can. We all miss the mark.*

Ramón shaves and washes and tidies the room in the low light of the desk lamp. He pulls the beige bedspread so taut that a dime would bounce off the surface, which is the way his father, an old soldier, had required it when inspecting his boyhood room. He stands back, and inspects the room himself, which looks as if no one is staying in it. All of Ramón's possessions are stowed in his travel bags in the closet, or in a ditty bag in a drawer by the sink.

The desk is clear except for his bible, his journal, and his pen. He sits upright on the chair, sit bones solidly in place, leaning into the light of the desk lamp. He opens his journal and his pen and turns to the scriptural passage that the Jesuit priest who is guiding his practice of the full Ignatian Exercises assigned last month. It is the Gospel of Luke, Chapter 15, which includes the parable of the prodigal son.

Ramón sighs. He can feel resistance already. He isn't accustomed to the New Jerusalem Bible, and he has read this parable so many times that he feels dry inside, and unsure of finding the narrow way. Drawing on his considerable discipline, he applies himself to the passage. Even though he knows it by heart, he won't rely on memory—he doesn't want to make a mistake. He is careful, diligent, and eager to put before God his best possible effort.

When he first attempted the full exercises eight years ago, Ramón gave himself a year, or four years, to master them, as if they were an internship or residency. Now he can see that they are the work of a lifetime, a slow catalyst for the wisdom of elders. When the practice is particularly slow, he uses it to develop patience.

Scanning the scripture, Ramón reminds himself that the prodigal son takes his inheritance, wastes it on liquor and prostitutes, and ends up in a distant land tending unclean animals. Famine comes, the prodigal son nearly starves, and finally resolves to return to his father and apply to be a servant. On seeing his son again, the father is overjoyed, and has his servants clothe the boy richly and prepare for him a feast. When the dutiful elder son comes home from the fields, he refuses to join in the feast, complaining that he never had such a reward for his years of good behavior. The father replies that the elder son is always with him and shares in all he has, and should rejoice at the return of one thought dead.

Ramón remembers when he first entered the parable as an observer at some distance, a servant, a guest at the feast and, after a time, when he was familiar with the scene, as the Prodigal Son.

This has always been easy for him, because he has turned away from the heavenly Father. In college, he avoided the Newman Center and joined a cadre of radicals eager to liberate the oppressed by force of arms. In medical school, he rarely attended Mass. Ramón could feel the Prodigal Son within him always, like a sentinel reminding him of St. Paul's call to unceasing prayer.

Unfortunately, Ramón has been like a man walking up the down escalator. He is making effort, but he seems to make no progress. He thinks wistfully of entering the scene as the father, in which case he would feel Godly love that is like a well of joy that never runs dry—but when he tries to do that, he instead feels like a green apple that should be left on the tree to ripen. But he has faith that someday he will feel that love, and then pass it on to others.

He should first enter the scene as the elder brother, but he has never been able to do that. He can't conceive of a brother showing uncharitable envy and judgment, anger and ingratitude, without at least a little amazement, relief, forgiveness, or joy. Ramón would feel all of that, even if his least favorite brother returned in shame, even if his family were Jewish and had treated the boy as dead and read the mourner's *Kaddish*.

Ramón closes his eyes and challenges himself. He will try again to enter the scene as the elder brother. He has never been to the Galilee, but he has seen pictures of it, which remind him of the village from which his grandfather came, and where he still goes to visit relatives. He takes pains to visualize it with clarity. When he can see the buildings, the father, the Prodigal Son, the servants, the trees, the paths, and the fatted calf on the fire, the tableau remains as still as a photograph.

He cannot find his way in. He cannot bring it to life. Casting about for ideas, he decides on impulse to rewind the elder brother's day. His body streaks a backward blur on an umber-tinged trail that has been worn by animals and their tenders into a white stone dotted hillside. Coming to a stop in a sloping field where the sheep are grazing, he grasps his twisted but smooth staff and uses it to drive them home.

He can't see Sepphoris, which is behind a hill on his right, but he is aware of the murderous and maniacal desire for power that gripped its tiny elite and turned them into predators. He is also aware of the greedy happiness felt, for the moment, by the builders and traders who serve that desire, some of whom were once members of his tribe. Those currents of feeling are nothing next to the distress of the Chosen who lost their patrimony to insatiable foreigners, whose repression pushes the tribe's rage into the land, where it simmers like a hidden hot spring.

These troubled thoughts are made more oppressive by the heat of the sun, which is well past its zenith yet still like a fire suspended just above his head. His water skin has been empty for some time. It has been so long since he drank of its warm water that only a lone trickle of sweat runs down his back into the dry rope around his robe. He has not passed water since noon. Once he has acknowledged his thirst, he can barely think of anything else. This frustrated desire becomes anger, which he transforms into the hard determination of a Pharisee. *Shiviti. I set the Lord always before me.*

The sheep are moving around each other like pebbles tumbling down the hillside. He would like to stop and remove the stones that have lodged in his sandals, but the sheep are moving too quickly. Perhaps they, too, feel thirst. The dust raised by their nimble feet penetrates the hem of his white robe. A gust ruffles the ears of his flock and covers his beard with fine powder. He looks gray, and feels like an old man.

Beginning to pray, and then to brood, he remembers when his father's household was a place of ease, and he could follow his heart's desire. Since fear and worry came into his life and into the lives of all his neighbors, his heart has been as hard as an overgrazed hillside of rocks and thorns. His only consolation is that his younger brother has disappeared, which means that he does not have to watch the boy fall ever deeper into debauchery.

He is still angry with his father, who did not restrain the boy's excesses. Their father's placid love was a sign of contemptible complacency. It tasted too much of sweetness, and too little of judgment. Becoming a Pharisee has made him bold enough to correct his father's weaknesses. He will do everything he can to keep the Covenant and observe the laws of Moses. If they all did so, God would lead all Yisrael out of servitude.

As his flock of sheep disappears around a bend in the trail, a long-bearded man in a dirty robe stumbles toward him, and then into him. He is gripped by fearful disgust. If the man is a foreigner, he has been polluted. He grabs the man by the arm, roughly, and demands to know if he is a Jew, and if he is observant. An exchange of words is enough to reassure him that he has not been polluted. The man is a righteous one; he is only distraught at the loss of his land and the rape of his wife by a Roman centurion.

The trail veers again, revealing a view of his father's house. It rises from the earth as if God himself raised it from the surrounding umber-tinted clay. He feels glad. His heart is like a withered fig tree with a few remaining fruits, one of which is affection for the God who has rewarded his righteousness by sparing the household of his father from violation and dislocation.

He notices immediately that something is wrong. The servants are scurrying about, and his father has killed the fatted calf as if for a last feast. He is gripped by a fear that some Roman official has finally come to claim their land, which should by rights be his inheritance, and without which they will all share in the fate of his prodigal, dissolute younger brother. Fear turns to puzzlement as he draws near enough to see that his father is receiving a guest.

Puzzlement turns to disbelief and condemnation when he draws close enough to see that the guest is his errant younger brother, who was rumored to be tending pigs, and whose presence is therefore a source of pollution and disgrace. He can hardly believe his eyes. As the sheep run ahead of him to the drinking trough, he lags behind, his eyes taking in more and more of the outrageous behavior of his weak-willed father. He sees now that the dead-to-Yisrael boy is wearing the best robe, and has a ring on one thorny finger and sandals on both pig-filthy feet.

He has never been so shamed and insulted, and for what? He has given years of faithful and righteous service to his father, but has never been so honored. For this disgraceful and disgraced son, his father even killed the fatted calf for a feast of welcome. He cannot bring himself to speak to his father at all, or to look at his good-as-dead brother.

As the vision lifts, Ramón feels the cold, hard desk under his elbows and becomes aware of the heat of the desk lamp. He is still somewhere between the world of the Bible and the world of today when he becomes aware that he is angry, ashamed, resentful, and full of blame and judgment. He feels an impulse to set the story right, to show whoever wrote the New Testament that the story is wrong, that the errant boy deserved one or more of the many punishments luridly depicted in the Old Testament—but the boy is already gone.

The feelings are still there, though, and seek a target the way a gun owner who has denied his buried blood lust too long feels an itch in his trigger finger. The reasons that he is right about his judgement line up in his mind like so many tin cans on a fence rail, and he finds his target immediately: Connie. He remembers the way she led him around the state on a merry chase, and then threw their protocols away; even having the impudence to assert her own judgment as to what was right and what was wrong. As Ramón comes fully awake, he finds that his fists are clenched.

Suddenly, Ramón recalls that he had seen the virtue in Connie's behavior the day before. Only a few hours before, in a meeting that had not yet seeped into the depths of his unconscious mind, he had forgiven her. In a flash, he sees the elder brother within. He sees that part of himself that climbs onto the throne of judgment that is not his, and which he should never presume to own. He feels a wave of shock and shame, and also a bloom of understanding and forgiveness for Connie, for the elder brother, and for himself. Later, when he is lying in bed, close to sleep, he sees that he has never been closer to putting on the mind of Christ. Gratitude opens the door to adoration; Ramón tastes the ecstasy of Divine Love.

Deep inside Ramón, in a place that medical science has not discovered—and will never understand—there is a fountain of tingling joy that gives way to the deep peace of knowing that he is truly seen and loved even in his errors. Peace pours from his heart, and he sends it into the world to those he knows and loves, to those he knows need it, and to all creation.

For the first time in years, the parable is alive in him again. He has sought new life assiduously and devoutly, and has recognized and received that grace opens him to holiness. He is so close to God in the glowing dark that he can't sleep.

Later, when he thinks of Connie again, he sees something

of Mary in her. He sees the incarnation mirrored in all women who are with child; and in all children who struggle into life.

He is blessed, deeply blessed, and renewed by his inclusion in the great Mercy that envelops all. Now he will notice the Prodigal Son within, and the elder brother within—and some day, when he is ready, he will see and be grateful for the father that is ever-present in himself.

15

Congregation

As Father Sean walks in, Mrs. Marino eyes him suspiciously. She is, as usual, sitting beside Mrs. Benettoni and holding the bent woman's hand. Father Sean, still flummoxed by Mrs. Marino's severity, decides to try an experiment. If she is trying to resurrect her earthly father who is gone, and no longer able to comfort her with stern certainty, she may feel better if Father Sean steps into the role of that kind of earthly father. He frowns darts at her, and is amazed to see her relax and allow a slight smile to warm her haughty regard for him. He can barely contain his surprise as his heart races to fill in the blanks: Her father may have been as severe as his, probably the type of hard man that, if he thought he needed to explain himself, would have said that to spare the rod is to spoil the child. He realizes in that moment that he must parent each parishioner differently, for the sake of his Father in heaven.

He adopts an air of solemn ceremony as he enters the confessional and listens carefully to what is and is not confessed. Near the end of the hour, Father Sean hears the sound of a voice that is becoming especially dear.

"Father Sean, I am troubled by many angry thoughts."

Father Sean looks at his watch, smooths his cassock, and remembers her first confession to him. He feels a twinge of regret at having fallen asleep both spiritually and literally, and recalls how much has happened since. He reminds himself to listen deeply.

"How many angry thoughts?"

Connie's complaints come pouring out in sorrow rather than anger. "I am angry that a priest violated my mother. That her parish punished her for it. That nuns taught me to believe motherhood belongs to abstinent virgins; that women, women's bodies, and fertility are evil. And that the miracle of new life is unholy until men have blessed it; that women deserve no goddess, no mysteries or rites for sex—even marital sex—or for fertility, procreation, or the bearing of children. And that, after all this, the Church claims that it is for life because it forbids abortion."

Connie's words spill like Communion wine that Father Sean is trying to put back in the cup. His mind seeks solid ground, torn between absolving, teaching, and fathering this child. He agrees with her, for the most part, and yet her words leave a stain in her, and in him.

"I am listening."

"*You* are not sick with a love of power or a hatred of women or life. How do you do it?"

"The miracles of the annunciation, the incarnation, and virgin birth are rich in meaning. It has been the aim of the church to prevent priests, and other men, from wronging women."

"Tell me, then, Father, that my thoughts are not evil." She begins to cry.

"You are not evil. You have never been evil. I could not love you like a daughter if you were evil." He puts his hand over his heart, which is flooded with pain that may be angina, or it may be heartbreak. He puts nitroglycerin under his tongue. It doesn't help. *Thank you Christ, for the gift of feeling.*

"Tell me that I am not an unwitting friend to inner death!"

"You are not unclean. You merit no punishment. Do not punish yourself—or others. Your penance is to accept me as your father in spirit and in life." *Please God, help me find the words.* "I ask you to accept my paternal love as it is, faults and all, and to invite that love to heal your wounds."

"Thank you, Father. I am so hurt and angry!"

Be angry and do not sin. "There is a holy anger, Connie, which comes of refusing to be overwhelmed by darkness. You have had more than your share of sorrow, and done more to alleviate the sorrows of others. Now it is time to put down your burden."

Father Sean clears his throat, then speaks with a bold intent that sounds unexpectedly hesitant. "May I give you some fatherly advice?"

"Yes, Father."

The word "Father" takes on a new tone, fraught with an uneasy mix of fear, love, and hope.

"When you feel strong emotions, take a break. Take the world off your shoulders. Sit in your easy chair and try to reconcile with the past, and to contemplate the future. Let the body of life through which we know the body of Christ reveal the true father that you seek. Let your unborn child, who is already a part of the body of life, teach you sweetness and love."

Connie sighs haltingly, and then says obediently, "I will, Father."

Father Sean is astonished at the number of people lined up outside the confessional, smiling eagerly at him, as if they had come to celebrate his visions. The buoyant mood seems to have affected everyone except Mrs. Marino, who is kneeling before the virgin but watching Father Sean through the black lace of her ample head covering, back twisted and shoulders tense. She may think that he is getting too easy on sinners, too reluctant to punish.

Father Sean looks sternly at Mrs. Marino, then enters the confessional eager to do God's work. He tells himself not to question the presence of so many penitents, and he doesn't, until after the fourth confession, which is followed by a strange request. "But Father, may I have your special blessing?"

After a long pause, he asks, "And what blessing, in particular, do you seek?"

"The blessing of the vision of the risen Christ. The blessing that Mrs. Hernandez and the Bishop received. Everyone's talking about it!"

"Ah," the priest sighs. Within seventy-two hours of his ride in the ambulance, the Bishop had sent over a Brother Gabriel from the Trappist monastery in Snowmass, who had been on his way home from giving a retreat in Colorado Springs. Brother Gabriel had filled Father Sean in on the lives of Meister Eckhart, Dame Julian of Norwich, St. John of the Cross, and Fr. Thomas Merton, of whom Father Sean had been only dimly aware.

And although Brother Gabriel positively glowed with the love of our Lord, the homilies that he gave in Father Sean's place used strange and unfamiliar words that frightened Mrs. Marino. And the Bishop sent Brother Gabriel home with the promise of sending Father Sean there on retreat. Even now, in advance of the retreat, Father Sean feels God's love in every moment, and embraces God's all-encompassing mystery, as if the world has been made new.

He intones warmly, "Blessing of the Risen Christ."

He ends each confession the same way, adding at the last,

"And the blessing of constancy in the name of our most constant worshipper, Mrs. Marino."

After this, he hears footsteps running across the apse and out the side door. He smiles, wondering whether she felt scandalized, or blessed, by the recognition.

Mrs. Hernandez edges closer and closer to Connie, and begins to stroke baby Rose's fine, downy, dark hair. As Connie suppresses a smile, she asks "Would you like to hold her?"

Mrs. Hernandez swoops in without hesitation and lifts baby Rose from Connie's arms. Although Connie's mother looks a little jealous, Mrs. Hernandez gives her a brief look, and a tip of the head, and the two women go off together.

Connie notices that Mrs. Hernandez is the only one who does not seem at all surprised, disappointed, or discouraged to find out that this episode of birth defects is to remain an unsolved mystery. To her, Connie realizes, all of life is a mystery—not just the Latin that she never understood, the communion wafers that transubstantiate in front of her eyes every time the Father says Mass, or the English words that elude her as if invisible lariats lasso them out of the air before they get to her ears. She knows that God knows, and she doesn't mind that she doesn't. It is as if she had known from birth that life and God will always defy human comprehension.

Connie looks around the rectory dining room, bright with sunlight streaming through the open curtains, and with the family and friends of the three infants who were just christened in the sanctuary. At the dark and heavy dining table, which adds gravitas to the sparkling clean crystal on the sideboard, Father Sean is telling Brother Ben about the latest exploits of the infants, including his god-daughter and god-granddaughter. Beside him, Pippie, who is at least 100 pounds lighter, is talking with Melissa and Dan.

Melissa catches Connie's eye, and, seeing that she is alone, comes briskly toward her. Then, taking the chair emptied by Mrs. Hernandez, puts a protective hand on her own swelling belly as she lets her thighs spread to make room for her unborn baby. If she sits like this, she will be comfortable for up to half an hour, perhaps more. The baby, who is kicking the place where huge red stretch marks have bloomed, has another foot on her bladder, which puts pressure on the tissue that makes her so crazy for sex that Dan has taken to hiding from her. She is looking forward to the evening, when she can lie on her side, heave her belly onto the body pillow, and free her pelvis and legs.

"My body has officially become unrecognizable. I'm an animal, not sure which one—too short to be a whale or elephant, maybe a small goat with bulging teats."

"Your breasts are huge, now!"

"Along with my ankles. But the breasts will be useful. I could photograph them and sell the pictures to puerile men, but I plan on saving them for the use God intended."

"The body's well designed, isn't it?" Connie remarks.

"Yes. And this one doesn't belong to me anymore. Nothing could be clearer. I'm just a way station, a stop on the road to life. Men can study women all they want, but they'll never know what it's like to be a woman. Never. No wonder they're frightened of us."

"We can't take our bodies that personally, can we? Mine belongs to Rose now, it will as long as I'm breastfeeding, and as long as I care for her and any children she may have. She gives me so much strength to love."

"Love *is* strength. And I suppose it doesn't hurt that you love your new life in the valley, or that Pippie is looking so much less like a risk factor," admires Melissa.

"Pippie loves me like crazy, and he's so supportive. Of course, I want him to be healthy, but I also want him to do what he wants. And I'm glad he's getting along with Dan so well."

"Pippie gets along with everyone." Melissa smiles. "He's like the stereotypical IT guy, isn't he? The organizational psychologist."

"Pippie isn't a stereotypical anything. That's one reason it's such a relief to go home to him. We live in a little world of our own in which we try to do as much good, and as little harm, as we can."

Melissa sighs. "Dan's a loner, as you know. I knew that he had little support as a child, and little challenge. It shows. But I'm beginning to see how helpless he is, and how much he craves love, yet fears it. He seems to be going deeper and deeper into his shell."

"He isn't like John," says Connie.

Melissa slumps and says sadly, "He's like John is now."

Connie looks at her friend sharply, and says with uncharacteristic tact, "It sounds like you're not over John."

"I never will be. John opened my heart the way Randall opened my body."

Connie retorts with a sweet laugh. "No, the way Dan did. That's his baby you're holding in there." She continues in a more comforting manner. "All of us are still who we were, deep down. You are; I am."

"Maybe. Maybe we only love once. In any case, it's better to love someone than no one."

Connie shifts to a confidential tone, changing the subject. "I'm surprised you decided to have a baby, given how aware you are of the toxic hazards that surround us."

Melissa sighs. "I am aware, but I'm also aware that it's safer now than at any time in the past. I can't imagine what it was like 100 years ago, when the mother and infant mortality rate was so high."

"I can't either. *And* I can't believe we didn't see these new risks before."

"I can. In college, I lived in a ghetto. I was afraid to go outside, and wasn't thinking about later. It's only now, when we're trying to realize LBJ's dream of the Great Society, that we can see the problems we've been creating." Shaking off her sadness, Melissa adds quietly, "It's wonderful to be able to see you more often, and to enjoy the love of other old friends from the Illinois and Oregon days."

"Yes, it is. And it's good to be home again. I do worry about the world we will leave our children, but thinking of you—and all our old friends—gives me hope that we will be able to leave our descendants a better world before we go."

Acknowledgments

For a world of education in the causes and consequences of epidemic diseases, I owe a debt of gratitude to the 1977 Clinical Pathophysiology Course of The University of Chicago; to Dr. Pierce Gardner for offering an independent study in Public Health; to Dr. David Silverstein for arranging student electives in Nairobi; and to the faculty, residents, staff, and patients of Kenyatta National Hospital for direct experience of global human affiliations. I owe an even greater debt to Drs. J. Thomas Grayston, Maureen Henderson, James L. Gale, and King K. Holmes for arranging a preventive medicine residency with a Master's program and employment in Public Health that enabled my board certification in the field; and to University of Washington Community Medicine affiliate Dr. Fernando Vega for setting an example for disease investigation through the practice of Family Medicine.

For an enriching education in multidisciplinary research collaboration, for the sharing of ethics, for public service, and for experience in outbreak investigation and the practice of Public Health in the context of environmental devastation, I thank my Colorado Department of Health and CDC colleagues from the bottom of my heart: Drs. Tom Vernon, Ellen Mangione, José Cordero, Dave Erickson, and Lois Freisleben. I would have understood nothing about the daunting task of peering into the unknown behind an emerging epidemic without your generous mentoring.

From the University of Colorado, I thank: methodologists David Savitz and Anna Barón; bioinformatics consultant Jessica Bondy; Dr. William Marine; medical anthropologist Lorna Moore; Dr. Dick Hamman of the San Luis Valley Diabetes Study; and my NIH project officer Dr. Alan Locke. I am also indebted to academics from elsewhere including Drs. Mervyn Susser, Paul Zimmet, Alvan Feinstein, David Sackett, and Elizabeth Barrett-Conner of the Society for Epidemiological Research.

Last and not least, I am grateful to the Southern Oregon team that made this book beautiful. The appearance is due to the professional competence and creativity of cover artist Bruce Bayard and book designer Chris Molé. The readability is due mainly to coach Chansonette Buck and editors Deidre Krupp, Deborah Mokma, Julia Anderson, and Ann DiSalvo.

Such writing ability as I am developing, I owe first to my father, who taught me reading and writing at a young age. I am also grateful to editor friends Eva Silverfine and Stephanie Holt for their talent and skill in verbal expression, to writing teachers Andrea Goldsmith of the Victorian Writer's Centre, and to Wendy Call of Hugo House. They kindly put up with an unusual and neurotoxic student, trusting that their wisdom would not go to waste.

Thank you also to my book development and beta readers, especially: Jan Agosti, Anna Barón, Jessica Bondy, Cynthia Bradley, Julie Clayton, Stephanie Holt, Christopher Howell, Joel Mason, Sara Myers Wade, Berta Nicol-Blades, and Dana Smaller. Special thanks to Jan, Anna, Julie, and Stephanie for their kindness in dark times.

About the Author

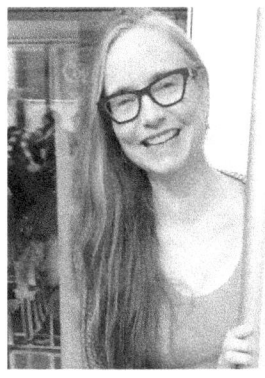

Beth Alderman, MD, MPH earned her AB and MD degrees from the University of Chicago and her MPH from the University of Washington. After Board Certification in Preventive Medicine and Public Health, she took a faculty position in the University of Colorado Medical School Department of Preventive Medicine, Biometrics, and Medical Informatics, where she did population-based epidemiological studies of adverse reproductive outcomes and methodological studies in clinical epidemiology. In her next faculty position at the University of Washington School of Public Health, she focused on risk factors for birth defects.

In 1996, she fell ill with the mysterious new plague and was given the provisional diagnosis "chronic fatigue syndrome". She has spent her time since studying her own case and pondering the reasons that her beloved profession failed her so completely. Fortunately, she discovered her cure, which may be of use to others suffering from one or more of the emerging epidemics affecting humans, their habitats, and life on earth.

For more about and from the author, see the following websites:

BethAldermanMD.com	*Free Information for all readers*
DoctorsOfLife.com	*For care and cure of all lives as one*
LivingFutureBooks.com	*Publishing Website*
LivingFutureCourses.com	*Educational Website with Free and advanced Courses*

Look for author's books on Amazon.com

Other Books by
Beth Alderman

Medical Phenomenology:
Chronic Ambient Poisoning

ISBN: 978-1-7332849-2-9

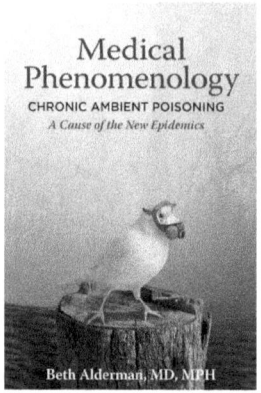

One day in December of 1996, the author (a physician, medical detective, and academic epidemiologist) developed disabling brain fog following on a decade-long descent into a painful, pervasive, and unprecedented chronic illness. Having done population-based studies to research the causes of birth defects, and having thus encountered the limitations of modern methods, she had inadvertently prepared to investigate the causes of her illness—which was given the provisional and uninformative label of "chronic fatigue."

The author began a delineation of the natural history of her condition using the methods of: doctors Hippocrates, Maimonides and Oliver Sacks; the "radical empiricism" used by Dr. William James; and the phenomenology introduced by Teilhard de Chardin and Merleau-Ponty. After a fifteen-year search, she found a doctor of integrative medicine whose elimination diet relieved her brain fog, which enabled her to complete a self-study and to construct an actionable new diagnosis: chronic ambient poisoning. Unseen by doctors and obscured by medical dogma and a myriad of false diagnoses, chronic ambient poisoning defies late modern, fragmented, accuracy-challenged medical research methods and delivery systems. It also reveals that human-caused habitat injuries that afflict birds, bees, and other species are affecting humans while driving evolved life toward extinction in the way of an asteroid strike. To ignore this diagnosis is to ignore the dangers to all lives posed by maladaptive modern lifeways.

The Evolve Fertility Series

BOOK 1
Melissa's Match: *Great Society*
ISBN: 978-1-7321110-1-1

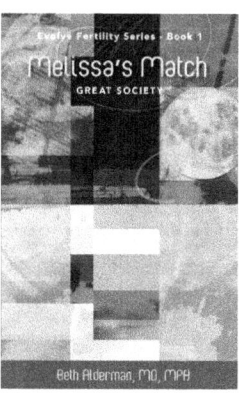

It's the early 1970s. Melissa and her friends begin their first year of college in the inner city of Chicago at a time when post-assassination riots, Great Society scholarship programs, and veterans returning from Vietnam create a sometimes explosive confluence of urban and rural, rich and poor, white and black, educated and uneducated. Coming of age in a violent, unjust, and yet hopeful time, they struggle to reconcile their hopes and opportunities with the shadows of war and the destructive clashes of senescing and emerging systems of care and cure of life on earth.

BOOK 2
Connie's Conception: *Awareness of Peril*
ISBN: 978-1-7321110-0-4

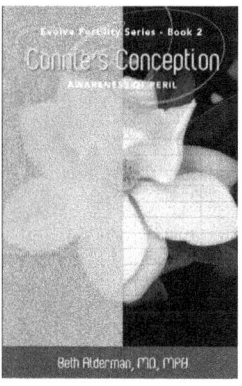

It's the late 1980s, and Connie Martin, a doctor working for the Epidemiology Intelligence Service of the CDC, is called to Colorado to investigate an alarming outbreak of birth defects. Born illegitimate in the San Luis Valley as Consuela Martín, a name known only to close friends and to her beloved gamer and programmer husband, she arrives as an unknown. Joined by environmental activists who suspect the state's Superfund sites and by doctors and parents who fear for its children, Connie attempts to discover the link between habitat destruction and damage to innocents.

BOOK 3
Melissa's Malady: *End of Modernity*
ISBN: 978-1-7321110-2-8

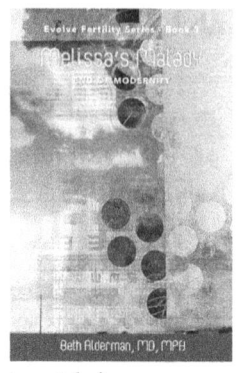

IIt is almost the year of the millennium, and Melissa meets her college friends Sarah and Doug and her first and only true love John for a reunion in Hyde Park. All four are in the midst of their careers. All struggle with the compromises that have marred their happiness. All wish to change the world, each in a different way. Sarah has left her government job for a new life as a yoga teacher. Doug is helping to birth a new value-based economy. John is a successful academic doctor. Melissa is ailing. They unite to turn John's success as a researcher to the cure of Melissa's mysterious chronic illness. What they find will change their lives and their imperiled world.

BOOK 4
Colette's Creativity: *Sacred and Profane*
ISBN: 978-1-7321110-3-5

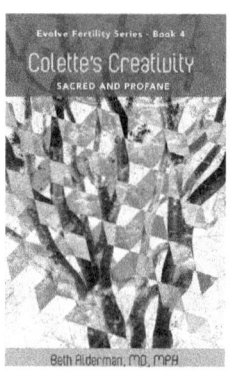

Colette, Melissa's childhood friend, abandons her marriage and home in Maine and flies to Melbourne. There she is taken in by her friend Reggie, who seems to know the secret of joy. Colette joins in the lives of striking individuals who lead her to view sexuality as a manifestation of the sacred. As she leaves behind the wounds caused by profane sexuality, she and her new friends clash with members of Reggie's family who force them to flee and to begin again.

BOOK 5
Colette's Community: *Thirds*
ISBN: 978-1-7321110-4-2

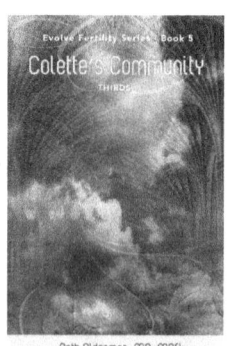

Soon after Colette and her friends find a new home, an old boyfriend of Melissa's who is sojourning in Australia calls and expresses his desire to visit. Colette plans to use the visit as a chance to develop a job for herself; he plans to check up on Colette for Melissa. As they get to know each other, they see that despite differences in religion, origin, and experience, they are on very similar spiritual paths. When it is time for Randall to go home, Colette joins him in Chicago. When he becomes caught up in his old life, however, she returns to Australia to pursue her dream of giving birth to a sacred community.

Chronic Illness Owner's Manuals

Regenerate Your Life: Chronic Illness as a Springboard for Creating Your Best Life

ISBN: 978-1-7321110-8-0 (VOL. 1)

ISBN: 978-1-7321110-9-7 (VOL. 2)

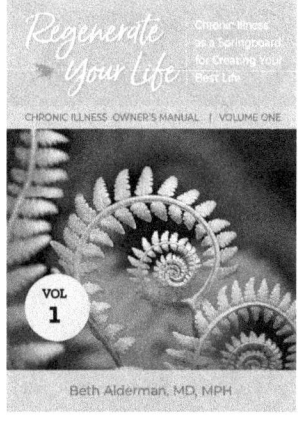

The *Chronic Illness Owner's Manual* series is for patients with chronic illness, and for the people who care for them. Suitable for individual or small group use, it offers a comprehensive, systematic, step-by-step approach to engaging modern medical systems, and to healing from the inside out.

The books comprise anecdotes, exercises, and quotes that address recovery through seven aspects of the body: awareness, understanding, perceptions, sensations, energy, flesh, and interbeing. The frames, constructs, patterns, and processes employed by the series are drawn from traditions of medicine, field biology, theology, and psychology from around the globe. Their synthesis offers an emerging, sustainable, eco-centric, eco-contextual, and customizable approach to creating a new and better life that regenerates your unique meaning, purpose, and vision of abundant life. The *Chronic Illness Owner's Manual* series complements care and cure courses available online at www. LivingFutureCourses.com.

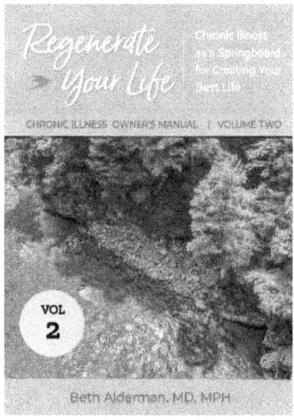

The Evolve Restoration Series
Sequel to the Evolve Fertility Series

BOOK 1
Pilgrim Minds: *After the War on Life*
ISBN: 978-1-7321110-5-9

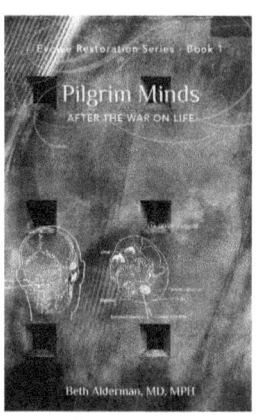

Melissa's deathbed request catapults her son Aaron on a journey from her family's Mississippian clinic to the Salish Sea to claim a mysterious legacy. Meeting his niece Rafa en route, he continues overland with her, and uncle and niece come to know and depend on each other. On arriving at the Saltspring Island Research Center (SIRC), Sarah, now the keeper of the center's narratives, confesses that Aaron's legacy is a task: to apply his mother's philosophy to SIRC's lifeways in order to revitalize it.

While he had been immersed in his mother's medical philosophy, SIRC had used many of her ideas to found a fertility school. SIRC's encroaching apathy persuaded Sarah that they missed one or more essential lifeways, and hopes that Aaron may be able to pinpoint and provide them. Taken by surprise, but ready to step up, Aaron immerses himself in the community, and Rafa undergoes SIRC's initiation process. Uncle and niece come to love Cascadia and to relish local, burgeoning patterns of innovation. Both choose to stay at SIRC, an agentic community that is doing much to restore evolution and its living future.

BOOK 2
Aaron's Legacy: *The Body of Life*
ISBN: 978-1-7321110-6-6

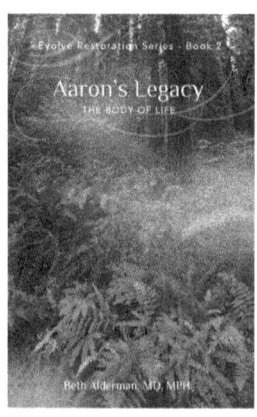

Having come to know the community, Aaron receives his legacy as a series of enactments of SIRC's history. The surviving members of his mother's old friendship group—Sarah, Doug, and John—join the audience and performers in processing and adapting their shared narrative. In the intervals between enactments, Rafa undergoes initiation while Aaron explores the composer, an instrument that enables a player to evoke memories with images and to express the player's responses as sound scapes. As Aaron shares his with Rafa, Sarah and others, John shares memories of Melissa, and seems to receive a new message from her.

As the community adapts to changes in its meaning and purpose, Rafa and Aaron each finds a first consort and draws inspiration from local knowledge keepers and change agents residing at SIRC, the nearby Monastery of Origins and Endings, or in Victoria or Vancouver. Aaron's health, damaged by his travel through a poison barren, deteriorates. With his death, his consort Parvati shares their legacy in the form of patterns of action that may remove roadblocks to continuous adaptation and renewal.

BOOK 3
The Kindred's Rebirth: *Rough Seas and Far Lands*
ISBN: 978-1-7332849-3-6

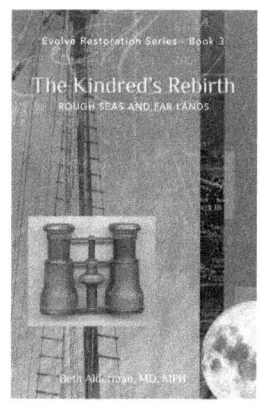

A decade later in Australia, Parvati and Björn give up on effecting meaningful restoration there. Dirk, while on his annual circuit of the north, arrives in Jokkmokk for the annual Sámi gathering to learn that SIRC is in crisis. Rafa, who is crossing the South Pacific on her two year global clinic circuit, hears strange news: the Fertility School, which was winding down, closed without notice. She realizes that her work, too, is drawing to a close as her clinics adapt to localism and begin to diverge.

All three travelers feel a strong homing urge and hatch a plan to converge in Scandinavia with the remnant of the SIRC community. En route, Parvati adopts a grandchild, Jacki, who helps Björn to recover from a disorder of interbeing. Many new consort pairs join the kindred and revive it by helping to form a next community, SIRC-Umea, and to organize and maintain residential restoration communities in the Baltic and North Sea bioregions, and to recover from the painful loss of the original community.

BOOK 4
Jacki's Vision: *The Green Line*
ISBN: 978-1-7332849-4-3

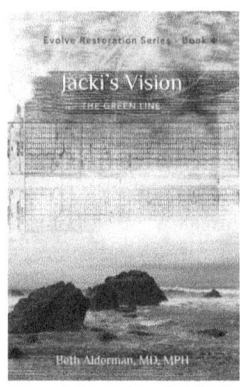

When Jacki turns sixteen, she begins her transition to adulthood by venturing into larger worlds of knowledge and adaptation to gain skills. During her first clinic circuit in the Baltic, she finds that her coming of age is coinciding with her kindred's restiveness. As she embraces and contemplates her future, a vision takes hold of her. She proposes a Green Line restoration project in Tasmania to reconcile a time debt created by the Black Line genocide, and to prepare her for organizing bioregional restoration projects. Her kindred and their networks embrace the project, expand it, and multiply its potential effects.

As the Green Line Corps prepares to depart en masse for Tasmania, Jacki meets a young stranger, Mirek, whose experience of the world—whose very umwelt—contrasts with her own. Later, in Tasmania, she gains a consort, Izaak, and a sister friend, Lally, both of whom winnow her possible futures. Together, the many thousands of Green Line participants develop a restoration ethos and synchronize living processes for restoring habitats—with their restorers. Jacki and her new peers are among the first to return to the original SIRC campus, near which many former kindred members have settled, and to which many others are about to return.

BOOK 5
Mel's Motherhood: *A Place in the Living World*
ISBN: 978-1-7332849-5-0

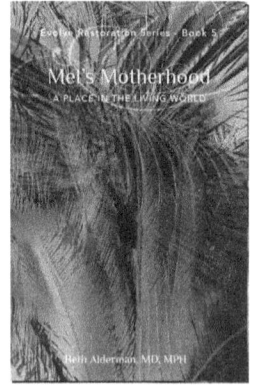

Mel and JJ—children of the Three Mammas—await the advance boat from Tasmania at the Cascadian Monastery of Origins and Endings. Mel, who is pregnant, and JJ, who fared poorly while he was away, finished their initiation projects and are keen to see Jacki and to meet the new kindred members. In the course of a joyful reunion, Mel and JJ learn that Jacki and Lally are also pregnant.

As this next generation of adults chooses ways to express fertility and defines new vocations, the reconstituting kindred celebrates new human lives, integrates with local communities, and processes hitherto hidden threads of SIRC's history with the aid of DNA fathers who participate. The complex, complementary communities adapt to continuous learning via phenomenology, and to continuous adaptation of systems for care and cure of evolved life.

Meaningful Retirement: *Become a Life Care Provider*

ISBN: 978-1-7332849-0-5

Meaningful Retirement is a self-guided monthly course in four seasons that can aid people like you who are exiting modern employment or withdrawing from the modern death economy. In it you will find a toolbox for transition to a vocation of life care, and thus begin to mature into a wise elder able to lead and mentor those who follow you. These seasons include:

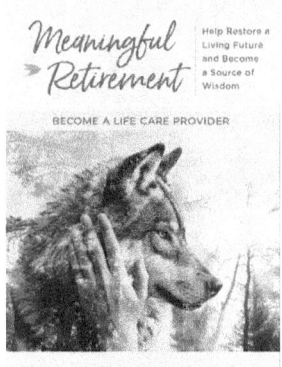

- **A Summer Breather**
- **A Fall for Reflection**
- **A Winter to Reclaim Your Personal Narrative**
- **A Spring for Revolutionizing Your Lifetime Learning**

As you transition to the role of provider of life care, you may choose to co-found emotionally and spiritually astute communities where you can mentor your juniors, who face the imminent and daunting task of passing through wrenching psychosocial change while arresting and reversing the accelerating human-caused Sixth Extinction. That threat to evolved life represents a unique crucible for transforming modern lifeways into ones that enable humans to choose and to restore life. Re-visioning and co-creating processes of care and cure that restore all lives as one will prepare your species to restore the planet's living lungs, its water circulation, its living shade, and its evolved resilience to unexpected planetary catastrophes. By viewing life in time though an eco-centric and eco-contextualized lens that scales from your lifetime to evolutionary time, you can begin to see your world through new eyes that reveal your place in the big picture of life on earth.

Direct learning, that is, phenomenology, is essential for restoration of a living future. This method has changed with every epoch since ancient natural historians began to attempt to create views, frames, and constructs in an attempt to grasp evolving generative systems. The present moment of peril can be taken as an impetus and inspiration to engage with an exciting process of learning and problem solving that some call the living paradigm. This paradigm, which is still incubating in fields as diverse as architecture and design, agriculture, archaeology, restoration, and theology, is ripe for grass roots syncreses across outdated fields of knowledge. When you learn to cooperate with the last hundreds of millions of years of evolution while pursuing space age ways of averting asteroid collision, you will be prepared to lead your species toward sustainability and to make room for rapid human adaptation that restores evolution. Welcome to the One Life..

www.ingramcontent.com/pod-product-compliance
Lightning Source LLC
Chambersburg PA
CBHW071518170626
46811CB00007B/2890